SIRTFOOD DIET

THIS BOOK INCLUDES:

SIRTFOOD DIET FOR BEGINNERS + COOKBOOK

MEGAN LEAN

THIS BOOK INCLUDES

BOOK 1: 10 (PAGE)

SIRTFOOD DIET FOR BEGINNERS:

A BEGINNER'S GUIDE FOR FAST WEIGHT LOSS. ACTIVATE METABOLISM, BOOST YOUR ENERGY AND LEARN A HEALTHY LIFESTYLE. INCLUDING A HEALTHY DIET PLAN

BOOK 2: 88 (PAGE)

SIRTFOOD DIET COOKBOOK:

SECRET RECIPES TO ACTIVATE METABOLISM, BURN FAT, BOOST YOUR ENERGY AND EAT HEALTHIER. A HEALTHY DIET PLAN FOR A FAST WEIGHT LOSS AND TO LEARN A HEALTHIER LIFESTYLE.

© Copyright 2020 - All rights reserved.

SIRTFOOD DIET FOR BEGINNERS:

A BEGINNER'S GUIDE FOR FAST WEIGHT LOSS.
ACTIVATE METABOLISM, BOOST YOUR ENERGY AND
LEARN A HEALTHY LIFESTYLE.
INCLUDING A HEALTHY DIET PLAN

MEGAN LEAN

TABLE OF CONTENTS

Introduction

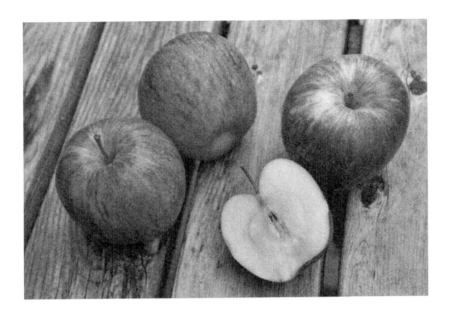

According to advocates, "Sirtfoods acts as an important regulator of our overall metabolism, primarily affecting fat burning while adding muscle and improving the physical shape of cells."

Burn fat, improve cellular capacity, and strengthen muscles: all these products are the exact products of the Sirtfood diet. Staying healthy and losing weight at the same time is the daily decision of every individual. You should take the first few steps and see how it can help you and your life.

If you want to take advantage of the beautiful results of Sirtfoods, here are some suggestions to start your diet:

Safety First- Always consult your health care professional before starting a diet or diet, especially if you have a current medical condition. It will ensure that the diet does not counteract any medication that you have taken or that has affected your health. Don't worry; the Sirtfood diet is pretty safe.

Knowledge Is Power- The diet is still very recent, but useful information is always available, and much remains to be done as this diet is rapidly gaining popularity. You can also search the Internet for recipes, food options, nutrients, etc.

Follow The Rules - Sirtfood is guaranteed to get results if you follow the recommended diet and meals closely.

Help Yourself - In addition to the requirements of the meal program, you can initially avoid processed and starchy foods from your healthy diet. Stop consuming garbage! This would accelerate the effect of the Sirtfood diet.

Start Physical Activity- the Sirtfood diet can burn these fats and help build muscle. Nevertheless, I advise you to include daily physical activities in your routine. Walking for 30 minutes a day would help your body and speed up the results. Also, there are beautiful effects in sport, for example, For example, preventing and fighting health problems that help improve your mood, burn calories, promote better sleep, give you boost energy, and more.

Go To The Supermarket -The Sirtfood diet only depends on certain foods. These foods have been collected for their ability to trigger sirtuin. So if you don't follow the grocery list, you won't see any results. Don't worry; I will provide you with a list of foods that are not too expensive and that you can easily find in almost any supermarket.

Put In Place the First "Restrictions" - If you want to get different results, you have to "sacrifice" a little to get the full result of the Sirtfood diet. Do not worry; the first three days are the most difficult for this diet because there are calorie restrictions. However, rest assured that every day is more comfortable. Although the restrictions imposed were not so strict for some who followed the diet, the reason was proper meal planning. You will not be hungry with the Sirtfood diet if you choose carefully.

Plan Your Meals Early Whatever your diet, planning your meals is a big help. Not only does this reduce eating stress, but you also can weigh your choices and fill your cupboard. You should keep track of the number of calories. You will be surprised that many filling dishes contain fewer calories and sirtuins.

Involve Your Dietary Partner- This diet can also benefit your family, your partner, or your friends (not only those who are overweight). It's also more convenient if you have a responsible partner who calls you back, shares recipes with others, or even cooks dishes with them.

Document Your Progress- You can start by taking photos and taking the required bodily measurements before starting the diet. You can also keep a food diary to monitor your food intake. Watch the changes in your body every week or phase. You can also have multiple goals to keep him alive and continue the diet.

Be Nice To Yourself - Don't set expectations too high. Yes, some can quickly lose up to 7 pounds in a week, but be aware that not all of our bodies are the same. And of course, your commitment counts. Other variables could be adding a workout plan to the diet plan, which could speed up the weight loss process.

CHAPTER 1:

What Is the Sirtfood Diet?

Sirt food is the latest trendy diet online after a famous singer like Adele lost 30 pounds by following the Sirtfood Diet. 2 celebrity nutritionists developed the sirtfood diet in the U k and since then gained a lot of popularity. Sirtfood diet is a diet rich in sirtuin activators. Sirtuins are a collection of 7 proteins that is responsible for balancing several functions in the body. This group of proteins is found in the body. It can also be increased through some natural plant compounds called polyphenols, consuming the kinds of nutrients in these plants can help elevate the amount of these sirtuins proteins in the body. Sirtuins are argued to promote cellular restoration and repair; they can also help balance your metabolism, burn fat, and boost muscle.

Who Came Up With The Sirtfood Diet?

Two health consultants and celebrity nutritionists Glen Matten and Aidan Goggins based in the UK wrote about The Sirtfood Diet. This diet concentrates more on a healthy eating pattern rather than just losing weight. This diet is divided into two-phase, you are expected to consume three sirtfood green juices and one sirtfood meal in this first phase and one sirtfood green juices with two sirtfood-balanced rich meals in phase two. The idea behind this revolutionary diet plan is that consuming this sirtfood juice and balanced sirtfood meal will help turn on your "skinny gene". According to the urban dictionary, "skinny gene" is a DNA sequence that predisposes a person to be thin regardless of the said person eating mass quantities of food and not working out.

How Do We Take Advantage Of Sirtuins?

So the big question is, how can we activate sirtuins and benefit from it? In general, we cannot but agree that exercise and fasting can help activate sirtuins in the body. But the only set back is that both can be very exhausting, having to maintain well followed through an exercise routine or food restriction. Exercise needs a lot of effort to effectively loss weight, while calories restriction can leave you feeling fatigued or cause muscle loss, irritability, hunger, and loss of stamina metabolic process; with these few shortcomings, achieving an overall goal might not be as easy as it sounds. Proteins belonging to the sirtuin family are helpful as anti-aging agents.

A research was carried out in 2013 between conventional modern diet and Mediterranean-style diet complemented with either nuts or extra-virgin olive oil. The reforms that were premised on the findings are called PREDIMED. The Mediterranean diet group showed slashed diabetes and heart disease by a massive 30 percent, with a significant reduction in risk associated with obesity. Although it did not come as a surprise, a further investigation carried out based on the general detail pointed out that both diets had no difference in calorie, carbohydrate, or fat intake. Amazing.

We are made to understand that there are natural compounds called polyphenols present in some plants that have enormous benefits for our health. The participant that consumed the highest amount of plants with these polyphenols within five years had 37 percent lesser deaths than the participant who ate the least.

Some of these selected polyphenols are capable of switching on our sirtuin genes without needing to exercise fast.

Although all Polyphenols are not the same, so will not give the same result when you consume them. Without any doubt, polyphenols help stay healthy and slim.

What Can Foods Activate Sirtuins?

With our overall knowledge about plants that contain polyphenols, serving as activation agent for sirtuin. Our whole interest is stimulated to get the highest amount of sirtuin-activating polyphenols incorporated into our diet.

This premise gave birth to the revolutionary Sirtfood Diet, a modern way of eating delicious foods while activating sirtuins. One good thing about Sirtfood Diet is you do not need to cut out carbs, eat low fat, or count calories. However, in the first phase, it is stated that combining sirtfoods with calorie restriction may activate the body to raise higher levels of sirtuins. Sirtfood Diet is characterized by eating the foods your love and still reaping the benefits of the diet. Now tell me, if you can eat what you love eating and even lose weight, is it not a diet worth embracing?

What Else Should You Eat?

You can combine the Sirtfoods with protein for a meal. Each meal can be accompanied with oily fish. To stress it out, moderate dairy consumption is perfectly okay".

It is good to understand that the Sirtfood diet does not concentrate on what not to eat; however, there is a need to avoid processed and sugary food or fish high in mercury.

Is This The Diet For You?

Any diet plan you adopt involves some level of expense and inconvenience. It may also involve risk. Anyone can write a diet, as there is no need to have the diet medically approved. That's one reason why all diets start by suggesting you consult a doctor. One thing you can do is look at the qualifications of the diet's author.

The authors of the sirtfood diet are not TV personalities or reality stars. They have genuine scientific knowledge of the subject, and both have Master's degrees to prove it.

Aidan Goggin is a pharmacist with a degree in pharmacy and a Master's degree in Nutritional Medicine. Glen Matten trained at the Institute for Optimum Nutrition before completing his Master's degree in nutritional medicine.

The sirtfood diet is not their first collaboration. In 2012, they wrote, "The Health Delusion," a that attacked many of the "long-held truths" of the diet and health industry. As a result, they received the consumer health of the year award by the Medical Journalists Association. Having the literature and asked the big question: "What would happen if we ate sirtfood? Would there be weight loss?" they went on to ask: "What would happen to muscle mass, which is usually lost during almost any diet?"
To find the answers, the authors conducted a trial in an exclusive health spa near London in the UK. There were 40 participants. 39 completed the test. Because the experiment was carried out at a health spa, the authors had complete control over the food eaten by the participants. Note that this is not always the case in "medical" trials where the participants report what they ate.

CHAPTER 2:

Pros and Cons of Sirtfood Diet

Pros

1. It Improves Powerful Exercise

Regular exercise is perhaps the best thing you can accomplish for your health and doing some direct exercise will improve the weight loss and medical advantages of Phase 1 of the diet. When in doubt, we urge you to proceed with your typical degree of activity and physical action through the initial seven days of the Sirtfood Diet. Be that as it may, we recommend remaining inside your typical safe place, since delayed or excessively extreme exercise may place a lot of weight on the body. Tune in to your body. There is no compelling reason to drive yourself to accomplish more exercise during Phase 1; let the Sirtfoods perform the complicated work.

2. It can be applied for underweight

A decent method to see whether you are underweight is to figure your weight file or BMI. For whatever length of time that you know your height and weight, you can, without much of a stretch, decide this by utilizing one of the various BMI adding machines on the web. If your BMI is 18.5 or less, we don't suggest that you leave on Phase 1 of the eating routine. On the off chance that your BMI is somewhere in the range of 18.5 and 20, we would look at present urge alert, since following the diet may imply that your BMI falls beneath 18.5. While numerous individuals seek to be super-thin, actually being underweight can adversely influence innumerable parts of health, adding to a brought down safe structure, a raised danger of osteoporosis (debilitating of the bones), and ripeness issues. While we don't suggest Phase 1 of the diet on the off chance that you are underweight, we do at present energize the combination of a lot of Sirtfoods into a decent method of eating with the goal that all the medical advantages of these foods can be harvested.

Be that as it may, if you are thin, however, have a BMI in the sound range (20–25); nothing is preventing you from the beginning. A larger part of the members engaged with the pilot preliminary had BMIs in the sound range yet still lost great weight measures and turned out to be progressively conditioned. Critically, a considerable lot of them announced a noteworthy improvement in energy levels, essentialness, and appearance. Recall that the Sirtfood Diet is tied in with advancing health as much as it's worth getting in shape.

Please, do not start the Sirtfood or any diet without medical advice and a physician following you.

3. Appropriate for weight loss

Being obese expands the danger of various constant medical issues, yet these are the very ailments that Sirtfoods help to secure against.

4. Provides Fiber

Numerous Sirtfoods are normally rich in fiber. Onions, garlic, and pecans are striking sources, with buckwheat and Medjool dates truly sticking out, implying that a Sirtfood-rich diet doesn't miss the mark in the fiber division. In any event, during Phase 1, when food utilization is decreased, the vast majority of us will, in any case, be eating a fiber amount we are utilized to, particularly on the off chance that we pick the plans that contain buckwheat, beans, and lentils from the menu choices. In any case, for others known to be powerless to stomach issues like obstruction without higher fiber admissions, during Phase 1, particularly Days 1 to 3, an appropriate fiber supplement can be thought of, which should be examined with your social insurance proficient.

5. Impacts may be within seven days

Seven days is what was tried and what is demonstrated to be viable. Be that as it may, if, for reasons unknown, you find that you have to stop it by a day or two, do as such by finishing up to the finish of Day 5 or Day 6. Try not to stress; you will, in any case, procure a lot of the advantages.

6. It very well may be natural and inorganic

Natural produce conveys a more extravagant substance of sirtuin-initiating supplements. Recall that the sirtuin-enacting polyphenols found in plant foods are created in light of natural anxieties. Without the exceptional utilization of pesticides, naturally developed produce should fight that a lot harder to prevent and avoid ecological predators. This is probably going to bring about more significant levels of polyphenols being delivered, making natural produce possibly a more impressive Sirtfood than its nonorganic proportionate. While natural is best, you will even now get extraordinary outcomes from the Sirtfood Diet if you decide on inorganic produce.

Cons

All diets have pros and cons—it's about finding the best fit for you. There is no need to eliminate a certain food group from your diet unless you have a medical reason to do so. Before trying a new diet, consider how it will affect all aspects of your life, including your social life and finances.

1. Ineffective With Medication

The Sirtfood Diet is reasonable for the vast majority, but since of its amazing impacts on fat burning and health, it can change certain sickness forms and the activities of drugs recommended by your doctor.

Discuss this diet with your doctor first before trying it. The odds are it will be fine and really of significant advantage for you, yet it's critical to check.

2. Can't be administered during pregnancy or breastfeeding

Try not to follow the Sirtfood Diet on the off chance that you are attempting to imagine or if you are pregnant or breastfeeding. It is a ground-breaking weight loss diet, which makes it objectionable. Notwithstanding, don't be put off eating a lot of Sirtfoods since these are astoundingly solid foods to incorporate as a major aspect of a reasonable and fluctuated diet for pregnancy. You will need to dodge red wine, because of its liquor substance, and cutoff energized things, for example, espresso, green tea, and cocoa so as not to surpass 200 milligrams for each day of caffeine during pregnancy (one cup of moment espresso contains typically around 100 milligrams of caffeine). Proposals are not to exceed four cups of green tea day by day and to maintain a strategic distance from matcha out and out. Other than that, you're allowed to receive the benefits of incorporating Sirtfoods in your diet.

3. Diet may cause mild symptoms

Phase 1 of the Sirtfood Diet gives amazing, normally happening food mixes in quantities that the vast majority would not get in their ordinary eating routine. Specific individuals can respond as they adjust to this sensational wholesome change. This can incorporate indications, such as a mild head-ache or tiredness, even though, as far as we can tell, these impacts are minor and fleeting.

If side effects are extreme or give you purpose behind concern, we suggest you look for clinical counsel. No different manifestations have never been seen other than incidental gentle side effects that resolve rapidly. Inside a couple of days, many people discover they have a restored feeling of energy, power, and health.

4. The Sirtfood diet is superfluously prohibitive; eating 1/200 calories daily is excessively prohibitive for some individuals

5. The diet likewise requires drinking up to three green juices for each day. Even though juices can be a decent wellspring of nutrients and minerals, they are also a wellspring of sugar and contain practically none of the solid fiber found in entire leafy foods

6. Tasting juice for the day is a poorly conceived notion for your glucose and teeth

7. The way that the diet is exceptionally restricted in calories and food deci-sions, it is more than likely inadequate in protein, nutrients, and minerals, particularly during the main stage.

8. There are some uncommon and costly fixings are the high beginning ex-penses of buying a juicer, just as the tedious costs of setting up specific meals and juices

9. Diet gets unworkable and unreasonable for some individuals. On the other hand, a diabetic individual, calorie limitation and utilization of juice during the primary days of the diet can prompt perilous changes in glucose levels

10. During the main stage, you may encounter opposite reactions, for ex-ample, weariness, tipsiness, and touchiness because of the calorie limitation.

CHAPTER 3:

Sirtuins

The sirtfood diet can't be classified as low-carb or low-fat. This diet is quite different from its many precursors while advocating many of the same things: the ingestion of fresh, plant-based foods. As the name implies, this is a sirtuin based diet, but what are sirtuins, and why have you never heard about them before?

There are seven sirtuin proteins – SIRT-1 to SIRT-71. They can be found throughout your cells and the cells of every animal on the planet. Sirtuins are found in almost every living organism and almost every part of the cell, controlling what goes on. Supplement Company, Elysium Health, likens the body's cells to an office with sirtuins acting as the CEO, For example, if a protein is available then the sirtuin can work with it to make something happen, just as the CEO can work with an available department head to make something happen. helping the cells react to internal and external changes. They govern what is done when it's done, and who does is.

Of the seven sirtuins, one works in your cell's cytoplasm, three in the cell's mitochondria, and another in the cell's nucleus. They have a full number of jobs to perform, but mostly they remove acetyl groups from other proteins. These acetyl groups signal that the protein they are attached to is available to perform its function. Sirtuins remove the available flag and get the protein ready to use.

Sirtuins sound pretty crucial to your body's normal function, so why is that you've never heard of them before?

The first sirtuin to be discovered was SIR2, a gene found in the 1970s which controlled the ability of fruit flies to mate. It wasn't until the 1990s that scientists discovered other similar proteins, in almost every form of life. Every organism had a different number of sirtuins – bacteria have one, and yeast has five. Experiments on mice show they have the same number as humans, seven. Sirtuins have been shown to prolong life in yeast and mice. There is, so far, no evidence of the same effect in human beings. However, these sirtuins are present in almost every form of life. Many scientists are hopeful that if organisms as far apart as yeast and mice can see the same effect from sirtuin activation, this may also extend to humans. In addition to sirtuins, our bodies need another substance called nicotinamide adenine dinucleotide for cells to function correctly. Elysium (see above) likens this substance to the money a company needs to keep operating. Like any CEO, a sirtuin can only keep the company working correctly if the cash flow is sufficient. NAD+ was first discovered in 1906. You get your supply of NAD+ from your diet by eating foods made up of the building blocks of NAD+.

The discovery and history of sirtuins

There were different quantities of sirtuins in every creature. For instance, yeast has five sirtuins, microscopic organisms have one, mice have seven, and people have seven.

The way that sirtuins were found across species implies they were "saved" with development. Qualities that are "rationed" have all-inclusive capacities in numerous or all species. However, what was at this point to be known was how significant sirtuins would end up being. In 1991, Elysium fellow benefactor and MIT scholar Leonard Guarantee, nearby alumni understudies Nick Austriaco and Brian Kennedy, led trials to all the more likely see how yeast matured. By some coincidence, Austriaco attempted to develop societies of different yeast strains from tests he had put away in his ice chest for quite a long time, which made a distressing domain for the strains. Just a portion of these strains could develop from here, yet Guarantee and his group identified an example: The pressures of yeast that endure the best in the cooler were likewise the longest-lived. This gave direction to Guarantee so he could concentrate exclusively on these long-living strains of yeast. This prompted the identification of SIR2 as a quality that advanced life span in yeast. It's critical to note more research is required on SIR2's belongings in people. The Guarantee lab consequently found that expelling SIR2 abbreviated yeast life range significantly. In particular, expanding the number of duplicates of the SIR2 quality from one to two grew the life length in yeast. In any case, what initiated SIR2 usually presently couldn't seem to be found?

This is the place acetyl bunches become possibly the most critical factor. It was at the first idea that SIR2 might be a deacetylating protein — which means it expelled those acetyl gatherings — from different atoms. Yet, nobody knew if this were valid since all endeavors to show this movement in a test tube demonstrated negative. Guarantee and his group had the option to find that SIR2 in yeast could deacetylate different proteins within sight of the coenzyme NAD+, nicotinamide adenine dinucleotide.

In Guarente's own words: "Without NAD+, SIR2 sits idle. That was the basic finding on the circular segment of sirtuin science."

Fun Facts about Sirtuins:

1. Mice that have been engineered to have high levels of SIRT-1 are both more active and leaner than normal, while mice that lack SIRT-1 altogether are fatter and more prone to various metabolic conditions.

2. Add the fact that levels of SIRT-1 are much lower in obese people than in those of a "healthy" weight, and the case for the importance of sirtuins in weight loss becomes compelling.

3. By making a permanent change to your diet and adding the best sirtfood to your eating plan, the authors of the sirtfood diet believe everyone can achieve better health, all without losing muscle mass.

To Sum Up

Exercise and calorie restriction are both sources of stress which encourage our bodies to adapt to changing circumstances. If the pressure becomes too high, the result can be an injury; the body can even die, but at lower levels, we adapt. This temporary, low-level stress is key to many physiological changes.

For example, stress on muscles, enough but not too much, makes the body increase muscle mass.

Similarly, the authors of the sirtfood diet found that when the body is stressed, by exercise or low-calorie intake, the effect of sirtuins kicks in, and this effect can be reproduced by a diet rich in SIRT foods.

CHAPTER 4:

Activation of Sirtuins

The Sirt Foods Diet is designed to activate sirtuins in the body. This is because Evidence suggests that sirtuins play a fundamental role in regulating circadian rhythm, oxidative stress, DNA repair, inflammation, cellular metabolism, tumour suppression and the stress response. They also inhibit fat storage and increase fat metabolism, thus potentially reducing the risk of diseases associated with excess fat including cardiovascular disease, some types of cancer, types 2 diabetes and arthritis. It is thought that these beneficial actions make sirtuins pivotal in regulating longevity and aging. With all these benefits you may be wondering how you can increase your levels of sirtuins. Read on to find out more!

Activation Of Sirtuins
What's really interesting is that the beneficial effects of sirtuins become activated during nutrient depletion, starvation and cellular stress, demonstrating that some physical stress on the body can be beneficial in small amounts (1?)

Molecules similar to sirtuins have been found in almost all species that have been studied including yeast, worms and fruit flies. Seven sirtuins have been identified in mammals with SIRT1 being the most widely researched. All Seven require NAD+, a derivative of vitamin B3 (niacin), to function. Niacin is found in mackerel, wild salmon, sardines, mushrooms, chicken, turkey, duck and whole grains (1).

Researched suggests possible ways to activated sirtuins include:

•Calorie restriction

•Physical activity

•Food components such as polyphenols and omega 3 fats

Our focus here is on the effects of Food on sirtuins activity but first let's take a quick look at Calorie Restriction and sirtuins.

Calorie Restriction and Lifespan

As SIRT1 increase when Food is scarce most researched into how to activated SIRT1 has focus on Calorie restriction (CR). CR has been shown to lead to extended lifespan in several species aging from yeast to dogs. The lifespan extension effects of CR has been strongly associated with a increase levels and activation of SIRT1. Intermittent fasting may also raise sirtuins (1).

The belief that many of the benefits of CR are due to the induction of sirtuins has led to researched into the sirtuins activating effects of foods.

Foods to Activate Sirtuins

Recent research has found that many of the foods and Food components that we know to be beneficial to health activated sirtuins in a similar ways to Calorie restriction. Here's the low down on sirtuins activating foods:

Resveratrol – is a polyphenols that has been shown to have a widely range of beneficial effects, including antioxidant, anti fungal, anti-inflammatory, anti-cancer and anti-mutagenic. It is now thought that some of the beneficial effects of Resveratrol are down to its ability to activated SIRT1 (2,3) although other mechanisms are likely to be at play as well. Resveratrol is found in berries, red grapes, peanuts, soy beans and pomegranate.

It should be noted that Resveratrol supplementation has been shown to blunt the beneficial effects of high intensity exercise on SIRT1 activation.

Quercetin – has been demonstrated to be a significant anti-inflammatory and anti-cancer agent that has protective properties against a number of diseases. These beneficial effects are partly due to the upregulating effects of Quercetin on SIRT1. Foods rich in Quercetin include capers, buckwheat, lovage, apples, tea, onions, citrus fruits, green vegetables and most berries.

Olive oil – a key components of the health promoting Mediterranean diet, olives and Olive oil are rich in beneficial polyphenols. Some of their health promoting effects can be attributed to their ability to activated sirtuins.

Cocoa or cacao is rich in flavanoids with many benefits particularly to cardiovascular health. Evidence suggests that some of their beneficial effects are due to the fact that they activate sirtuins.

Green tea – contains epigallactins that upregulate sirtuins.

Piceatannol – a naturally occurring analogue of Resveratrol, its displays antioxidative, anti-tumour and anti-inflammatory activities that may be due to its activation of sirtuins. Its is found in various plants, including grapes, passion fruit, white tea, and Japanese knotweed.

Green vegetables – Indole-3-carbinol (I3C), found in Brassica vegetables such as broccoli and cabbage, has powerful anti-cancer properties. I3C has also been found to ameliorate adiopogenesis (fat formulation) by activating sirtuins, making it a possible anti-obesity agent.

Turmeric – a rich source of curcumin that has been shown to exhibit many anti-inflammatory and neuroprotective effects which are partly down to activation of SIRT1.

Soy foods – contains isoflavones with many reported health benefits some of which may be attributed to the activation of SIRT1 signaling. Good source of isoflavones include tofu, tempeh and miso.

Omega 3 fats – Several studies have shown that omega-3 fatty acids can improve cardiovascular health, inflammation, insulin sensitivity and autoimmune disorders. This may be partly due to their effects on SIRT1 activation.

Melatonin – known as the sleep hormone due to its association with the circadian rhythm, Melatonin is also a powerful antioxidant and anti-inflammatory. Levels of melatonin tend to decline with age and its loss contributes to some of the degenerative conditions of aging. Evidence suggests that melatonin activates sirtuins.

A Note of Caution
There is some question as to whether the effects of these compounds on sirtuins in animals in laboratory conditions can be extrapolated to humans (15). Also much of the research into the activation of sirtuins has focused on supplemental levels of polyphenols which are much greater than would be found in Food. Future research is source to provide further insight into the role of foods and sirtuins in health and longevity as well as discovering many more biological mechanisms that affect body function. It the many time it seems there is sufficient Evidence to include these nutrient rich foods in the diet to support many aspects of health be it through their effects on sirtuins or not.

A Diet To Activate Sirtuins and Promote Health

Its probably no coincidence that some of the longest lived and healthiest populations in the world eat diets that are rich in these sirtuins activating foods, such as those in the Mediterranean and parts of Asia. The Mediterranean diet includes polyphenol rich fruits, vegetables, red wine and Olive oil. The Asian diet is high in isoflavones from soya beans and epigallactins from green tea.

A Successful Stories of Sirtfood Diet is the Famous Singer Adele blinds her beautiful voice millions of times, people in her photos speak of current opportunities! The 31-year-old woman looks thinner and fitter than before and is looking for inspiration!

Finally, imagine a scenario in which we will let you know that the success of Adèle's change is to eat brilliantly. As a fan of the "Sirt Food Diet", Adele followed this diet to lose weight and take a more beneficial and (obviously excellent) form.

Getting more of these health promoting foods into your diet is relatively easy. They can be incorporated into many meals and even combined to make super-sirt meals!

Here are some ideas to get you started:

•Use Olive oil for stir frying or roasting vegetables and salad dressings.

•Have a jar of olives handy to snack on and add olives to salads or cooked dishes. Tapenade makes a Good topping for oat cakes or rye bread.

•Swap regular tea and coffee for green tea. Add a squeeze of lemon for extra benefits.

•Miso can be used instead of stock cubes to flavour soups, stews and casseroles. Milder light coloured miso can be used as a spread. Miso soup makes a Good snack or light meal if served with salad or bread.

•Add tofu or tempeh to stir fries. Blend silken tofu into soups, dips and creamy desserts.

•Add berries and blackcurrants to muesli, smoothies and juices. Naturally yoghurt with fresh berries makes a health snack or desserts.

•Eat your greens. Kale, cabbage and broccoli are excellent accompaniments to any meal and can also be added to stir fries, curries, stews and casseroles.

•Spice up your life with Turmeric and other species. Don't limit your Use of species to curries; add them to grains and vegetables as well.

•Add cacao powder to smoothies and desserts. Sprinkle cacao nibs into salads or add to trail mixes.

•Apples are the perfect portable snack. Have one with you at all times.

•Buckwheat pasta can be used as a tasty gluten free alternative to wheat pasta and buckwheat flour can be used in baked goods or to thicken sauces. Buckwheat also works well in salads mixed with roasted vegetables and toasted nuts.

CHAPTER 5:

How Sirtfoods Helps To Burn Fat

Ecological factors significantly influence living beings' destiny, and sustenance is one of the most persuasive variables. These days life span is a significant objective of medicinal science and has consistently been a fabrication for the individual since antiquated occasions. Precisely, endeavors are planned for accomplishing effective maturing, to be specific a long life without genuine ailments, with a decent degree of physical and mental autonomy and satisfactory social connections.

Gathering information unmistakably exhibits that it is conceivable to impact the indications of maturing. Without a doubt, wholesome mediations can advance wellbeing and life span. A tribute must be given to Ansel Keys, who was the first to provide strong logical proof about sustenance's job in the wellbeing/sickness balance at the populace level, explicitly in connection to cardiovascular illness's primary source of death overall. It is commonly valued that the sort of diet can significantly impact the quality and amount of life, and the Mediterranean eating regimen is paradigmatic of an advantageous dietary example.

The developing cognizance of the beneficial impacts of a particular dietary example on wellbeing and life span in the second 50% of the only remaining century produced a ground-breaking push toward structuring eats fewer carbs that could diminish the danger of constant maladies, subsequently bringing about solid maturing. Subsequently, during the 1990s, the Dietary Approaches to Stop Hypertension (DASH) diet was contrived to assess whether it was conceivable to treat hypertension, not pharmacologically. To be sure, the DASH diet was like the Mediterranean Diet, being wealthy in foods grown from the ground, entire grains, and strands, while poor in creature-soaked fats and cholesterol. The excellent news leaving the investigation was that not exclusively did the DASH diet lower circulatory strain; however, it additionally diminished the danger of cardiovascular infection, type 2 diabetes, a few sorts of malignant growth, and other maturing related maladies To additionally improve the medical advantages of plant nourishment rich, creature fat-terrible eating routines, especially in hypercholesterolemia people, the Portfolio Diet was planned This eating regimen, other than being to a great extent veggie-lover, with just limited quantities of saturated fats, prescribes a high admission of utilitarian nourishments, including thick filaments, plant stanols, soy proteins, and almonds likewise. Curiously, members on the Portfolio Diet displayed a decrease of coronary illness chance related to lower plasma cholesterol and incendiary files compared with members on a sound, for the most part, vegan diet.

Nonetheless, additionally, the measure of ingested nourishment has been pulling in light of a legitimate concern for mainstream researchers as a potential modifier of the harmony among wellbeing and infection in a wide range of living species. Specifically, calorie limitation (CR) has been exhibited as a rising healthful intercession that animates the counter maturing instruments in the body.

In this way, the eating routine of the individuals living on the Japanese island of Okinawa has been widely broken down on the grounds that these islanders are notable for their life span and expanded wellbeing range, bringing about the best recurrence of centenarians on the planet. Interestingly, the customary Okinawan diet came about to be fundamentally the same as the Mediterranean Diet and the DASH diet regarding nourishment types. Be that as it may, the vitality admission of Okinawans, at the hour of the underlying logical perceptions, was about 20% lower than the standard vitality admission of the Japanese, along these lines deciding an average state of CR.

 In his most recent examination, showing up in the Aug8 print release of the diary Cell Metabolism, he saw what happens when the SIRT1 protein is absent from fat cells, which make up muscle versus fat.

When putting on a high-fat eating regimen, mice coming up short on the protein began to create metabolic issues, for example, diabetes, much sooner than typical mice were given a high-fat eating routine.

"You've expelled one of the protections against metabolic decay, so on the off chance that you presently give them the trigger of a high-fat eating routine, they're considerably more delicate than the typical mouse."

The discovery raises the likelihood that medications that upgrade SIRT1 action may help ensure against weight connected illnesses. From that point forward, these proteins have been appeared to arrange an assortment of hormonal systems, administrative proteins, and different qualities, keeping cells alive and solid.

Their past work has uncovered that in mind, SIRT1 ensures against the neurodegeneration seen in Alzheimer's, Huntington's, and Parkinson's ailments.

SIRT1 is a protein that expels acetyl bunches from different proteins, changing their movement. The potential focuses of this deacetylation are various, which is likely what gives SIRT1 its full scope of defensive forces, Guarantee says.

In the Cell Metabolism study, the specialists investigated the several qualities that were turned on in mice lacking SIRT1 yet encouraged a typical eating regimen. They found that they were practically indistinguishable from those turned on in ordinary mice sustained a high-fat eating regimen.

This recommends in typical mice, improvement of the metabolic issue is a two-advance procedure. "The initial step is inactivation of SIRT1 by the high-fat eating routine, and the subsequent advance is all the terrible things that follow that," Guarantee says. The scientists explored how this happens and found that in ordinary mice given a high-fat eating routine, the SIRT1 protein is cut by a compound called caspase-1, which is instigated by irritation. It's now realized that high-fat eating regimens can incite irritation. However, it's hazy precisely how that occurs, Guarantee says. "What our examination says is that once you incite the fiery reaction, the fat cells' outcome is that SIRT1 will be severed," he says.

That is discovering "gives a pleasant sub-atomic system to see how fiery signals in fat tissue could prompt quick unhinging of metabolic tissue," says Anthony Suave, a partner teacher of pharmacology at Weill Cornell Medical College, who was not part of the exploration group.

Medications that focus on that incendiary procedure, just as medications that improve sirtuin action, may have some gainful remedial impact against heftiness related issues, Suave says.

CHAPTER 6:

Masters of Muscles

One surprising result from our pilot trial that puzzled us was that the participants' muscle mass did not drop; instead, it rose by just over 1 pound on average. While it was common to see weight loss on the scales of 7 pounds, we saw something fascinating. The injuries on the levels initially appeared more disappointing than this for almost two-thirds of our participants, though still very impressive, with a weight loss of just over 5 pounds. But when tests were done on body composition, we were astonished. In these participants, muscle mass was not only maintained; it had increased. The total muscle benefit for this category was almost 2 pounds, adding 7 pounds to a "muscle gain-based weight loss."

This was unexpected and in stark contrast to what is typically the case for diets for weight loss, where people lose some fat but also lose muscle. For any diet which limits calories, it's the classic trade-off: you kiss good-bye muscle as well as fat. This is not surprising when you consider that cells change from growth mode to survival mode as we rob the body of nutrition and use the protein from the muscle as food.

What's good about maintaining Muscles?
So, what's that big deal? Do you know? Firstly, that means you're going to look much better. Stripping away weight while maintaining muscle leads to a healthy, toned, and competitive body that is more attractive. And more specifically, you should remain good looking. The skeletal muscle is the main factor that accounts for our body's daily energy output, which ensures the more muscle you have, the more calories you use, even when you rest. This helps support further weight loss and increases the likelihood of long-term success. As we now learn, weight loss with typical diet results from both fat loss and muscle loss, and thereby we see a marked decline in the metabolic rate. This induces the body to regain weight once more regular eating habits are resumed. But you burn fatter with a minimal drop in metabolic rate by holding your muscle mass with Sirtfood. This provides the perfect basis for weight-loss success over the long term.

In addition, muscle mass and function are predictors of well-being and healthy aging. Maintaining the muscle prevents the development of chronic diseases such as diabetes and osteoporosis, as well as keeping us mobile into older age. Importantly, it also seems to make us happy, with scientists believing that even the way sirtuins retain muscle has implications for stress-related disorders, including depression reduction.

All in all, weight loss when maintaining the body is a biggie and an even more desirable outcome. It's a unique feature of the Sirtfood Diet, and we need to get back to the sirtuins, so their substantial impact on the muscle to understand why better.

Sirtuins and Muscles Mass

In the body, there is a family of genes that function as guardians of our muscle and, when under stress, avoid its breakdown: the sirtuins. SIRT is a potent Muscle Breakdown Inhibitor. As long as SIRT is activated, even when we are fasting, muscle breakdown is prevented, and we continue to burn fat for fuel.

But SIRT's benefits aren't ending with preserving muscle mass. The sirtuins work to increase our skeletal muscle mass. We need to delve into the exciting world of stem cells and illustrate how that process functions. Our muscle comprises a particular type of stem cell called a satellite cell that regulates its development and regeneration. Satellite cells sit quietly most of the time, but they are activated when a muscle gets damaged or stressed. By things like weight training, this is how our muscles grow stronger. SIRT is essential for activating satellite cells, and without its activity, muscles are significantly smaller because they no longer have the capacity to develop or regenerate properly.6 However, by increasing SIRT activity, we boost our satellite cells, which encourage muscle growth and recovery.

Sirtfood versus Fasting

This leads to a big question: if activation of the sirtuin increases muscle mass, why do we lose muscle when we fast? Fasting also stimulates our sirtuin genes, after all. And therein is one of the fasting's big pitfalls.

Stay with us as we dig into the mechanics of this. Not all skeletal muscles are created equal to each other. We have two main types, named type-1 and type-2, conveniently. Type-1 tissue is used for longer duration movements, while the type-2 muscle is used for short bursts of more intense activity. And here's where it gets intriguing: fasting only increases SIRT activity in type-

1 muscle fibers, not type-2, so type-1 muscle fiber size is maintained and even noticeably increases when we fast. Sadly, in complete contrast to what happens in type-1 fibers during fasting, SIRT rapidly decreases in type-2 fibers. This means that fat burning slows down, and muscle breaks down to provide fuel, instead.

But fasting for the muscles is a double-edged sword, with our type-2 fibers taking a hit. Type-2 fibers form the bulk of our concept of muscle. So even though our type-1 fiber mass is growing, with fasting, we still see a substantial overall loss of muscle. If we were able to stop the breakup, it would make us look aesthetically healthy and help promote more loss of weight. The way to do this is to combat the decrease in SIRT in muscle fiber type-2 caused by fasting.

Researchers at Harvard Medical School tested this in an elegant mice study. They showed that the signals for muscle breakdown were switched off by stimulating SIRT activity in type-2 fibers during fasting, and no muscle loss occurred. The researchers then went to one step forward and checked the effects of increased SIRT behavior on the muscle while feeding the mice instead of fasted, and found it triggered a very rapid growth of the muscle. Within a week, muscle fibers with increased SIRT activity showed an amazing weight gain of 20 percent.

These findings are very similar to the outcome of our Sirtfood Diet trial, though, in effect, our study has been milder. By increasing SIRT activity by eating a diet rich in sirtfood, most participants had no muscle loss— and for many, it was only a moderate fast, muscle mass that increased.

Keeping Muscles Young
And that is not just the thickness of the body. SIRT's prolific effects on the muscle extend to the way it works too. As the muscle ages, it loses the ability to activate SIRT. This makes it less sensitive to exercise benefits and more vulnerable to free radicals and inflammation destruction, resulting in what is known as oxidative stress. Gradually muscles wither, become softer, and fatigue faster. But if we can increase SIRT activation, we can stop the decline associated with aging.

Indeed, by activating SIRT to stop the loss of muscle mass and function we usually see with aging, we see multiple related health benefits, including the halting of bone loss and prevention of increased chronic systemic inflammation (known as inflaming), as well as improvements in mobility and overall quality of life. So, interestingly, the latest research indicates that the higher the polyphenol level (and thus sirtuin-activating nutrients) in older people's diets, the higher the security they enjoy against deteriorating physical performance with age.

Don't be fooled into thinking that those incentives extend only to the elderly, far from that. By the age of twenty-five, the signs of aging will begin, and the muscle gradually erodes, with 10 percent loss of muscle around age forty (although overall weight tends to increase) and a loss of 40 percent by ages seventy. Yet there is growing evidence that the activation of our sirtuin genes will inhibit and reverse all of this.

Loss of muscle, development, and function: sirtuin behavior plays a crucial role in all of this. Stack it up, and it's no surprise that sirtuins were identified as master regulators of muscle growth in a recent in the prestigious medical journal Nature, with growing sirtuin activation cited as one of the promising new avenues for combating muscle loss, thereby increasing the quality of life, as well as reducing disease and death.

Looking at the powerful effects our sirtuin genes can have on the muscles, our pilot trial's shock results no longer seemed so shocking. We started to realize that driving weight loss when feeding our muscles was achievable through a diet rich in Sirtfood.

But it's just the beginning. we'll see Sirtfood' benefits extending so much too all aspects of health and quality of life.

CHAPTER 7:

Who Should Try The Sirtfood Diet?

Anyone who can make the best use out of this diet should try it. There is no one formula of who should try the sirtfood diet and who shouldn't. However, based on the body's needs and the physical problems a person is suffering from, we can decide on a better utility of this diet. The following are the cases in which the sirtfood diet can prove to be most effective.

1. Obesity
Sirtuin burns fats quickly, and that's what makes this diet a great help for weight loss. When we study all the cases of the successful sirtfood dieters, we can see how well they fought against obesity. Adele is just one example, who has amazed the world with her 30 pounds of weight loss achievement using the sirtfood diet. So, anyone who is not able to lose some extra pounds for whatever reason, they can switch to sirtfood and then can see the magic happening.

2. Low or Poor Metabolic Activity
Since sirtuins are mainly responsible for better cell metabolism, lower sirtuin levels in the body can hamper the natural cell activities and hinders the metabolism. Poor metabolic activity results in weakening of physical strength, obesity, hormonal imbalance, low enzymic activity, and several other related problems. The sirtfood diet is therefore suggested to boost the metabolic rates in the body and revitalize the body and the mind with levels of energy.

3. No workouts
Extraneous workouts are just not for everybody. Sure, working out is a good way to lose some pounds, but every other person can't invest the required time and energy into the workouts. Therefore, the sirtfood diet can be used by such individuals. Through this diet, they can manage their weight and lose it even while doing some basic physical activities.

4. Aging
Aging seems like a threat to all when those wrinkles start appearing on the skin, and the person feels weakened inside out! Well, this magic gene sirtuin

can also play its part in countering the effects of aging. It helps DNA to prolong its life and also aid in the repair process. Sirtuin is also responsible for apoptosis and leads to the formation of new healthy cells. This is the reason that people who are entering into middle age should consider doing the sirtfood diet so that they could effectively fight the possible signs of aging in the years to come.

5. Inflammation

What appears to be weight gain or metabolic inactivity is mostly connected to inflammation of both cells and organs in most cases. This inflammation is both the result and cause of several health problems. Sirtfood does not only prevent inflammation at cellular levels but effectively prevents it at the tissue and organ level.

6. Stress

There is one added advantage that higher sirtuin levels can guarantee, and that is the reduction in stress and depression. Research is still being conducted on the relationship between sirtfood and stress, but sirtuin is that element that can enable quick brain cell recovery and boosts brain activity by getting rid of all the unwanted metabolic waste. Efficient brain functioning then leads to a reduction in stress. So, this sirtfood diet can also help with stress relief.

The Procedure of the Sirtfood Diet

One step at a time! That's what it takes to incorporate sirtfood into your diet. The diet is simple and easy to follow in a sense that it only calls for a few definite steps to take. Firstly, you will need to increase food consumption that is rich in sirtuin, then you will have to follow the phases of the diet, plus you will need to add green juices to your daily diet. Here are a couple of steps that must be followed to achieve your weight loss goals on a sirtfood diet:

1. Get the right ingredients

Remember that all this diet asks from you is to increase your sirtuins intake. That can be done only through careful and selective grocery shopping. Prepare a list of the ingredients that contain a high amount of sirtuins and check their utility as per your meal plan. There are certain ingredients like coffee, parsley, red wine, and chocolate that you can have all the time. So, stock up your kitchen cabinets with these ingredients.

2. Set up the schedule

The sirtfood diet gives you small weight loss targets for each week. In the initial period, you must prepare a schedule to keep track of your meals, the caloric intake, and the timing of green juices you are consuming in a day. In this way, you will be able to manage the first few days of the diet adoption easily and continue observing body changes and measure your weight to keep track of your pace.

3. Prepare for the first week

In the first week of the sirtfood diet, the dieter must control his caloric intake. Therefore, to avoid any mistakes or confusion, all the high caloric food items should be removed from sight. Stuff your refrigerator only with the food that is appropriate for the sirtfood diet, and keep the juices, fruits, and vegetables ready to use. Instead of planning your meal every other day, make plans for the entire week according to the caloric limitations.

4. Caloric intake

Keep in mind that sirtfood is more about weight loss, so mere sirtuins cannot magically work overnight if you keep consuming more calories than your body can burn. Do the math and understand your caloric needs, even when the diet does not restrict you from high caloric intake after the first seven days. Still, you must maintain a strict check on the daily caloric intake to keep the weight in control. Otherwise, it does not take much to regain the lost pounds.

5. Green juices

Green juices are one of the essential parts of the sirtfood diet. These are your way to detoxification and quick weight loss. Green veggies are full of phytonutrients, minerals, and antioxidants. Having them frequently throughout the day can help boost the metabolism, remove the metabolic waste from the body, and enables the body to metabolize the needed nutrients appropriately. These juices are also great for keeping electrolyte balance in the body.

6. Maintenance

To harness the benefit of this diet or any other diet for that matter, it is imperative to maintain your new dietary routine. Most people abandon the diet as soon as they are an oven with the first two phases of the diet or when they achieve their weight loss goals. And soon, they regain weight and blame the diet for being ineffective, which is far from true. It all depends on how consistently you follow this diet plan.

Foods to Enjoy		Foods to Avoid
Vegetables		**Vegetables**
Kale	String	Nightshades such as
Beans		Banana Peppers
		Chili Peppers

Spinach Water Chestnut Collards Cauliflower Arugula Fennel Broccoli Lettuce Carrots Peppers Cabbage Rhubarb Artichoke Shallots Asparagus Mushrooms Beets Garlic Brussel SproutsOnion Zucchini Leeks Squash Radishes Watercress Chard BeetsBok Choy Celery Cucumber Turnips **Fruits** Apple Blueberries Watermelon Pomegranate Apricot Cantaloupe Banana Plum Strawberries Pineapple Blackberries Cherries Starfruit Pear Dates Papaya Figs Orange Nectarine Grapes Mango Guava Lemon Honeydew Kiwi Clementine	Thai Peppers Tomatoes Tomatillos Pimentos Sweet Peppers Habanero Eggplant Jalapeno Potatoes (sweet potatoes are ok) Artichoke All canned and frozen vegetables should be avoided. **Fruits** All canned and frozen fruits should be avoided.
Vegetarian Protein Tempeh Soy Nuts Edamame Soy Milk Tofu Organic Eggs	**Vegetarian Protein** Dairy Frozen or processed meals Nonorganic eggs
Protein Tuna Flounder Clams Shrimp Striped Bass Rainbow Trout Snapper Sardines	**Protein** Red meat with hormones Processed meats such as deli meat, hot dogs, bacon, and sausage.

Crab Halibut Herring Salmon Lobster Oysters Skinless Chicken Organic Eggs	
Grains Barley Black Rice Wild Rice Quinoa Brown Rice Oats Buckwheat Millet Bulgar Farro Corn	**Grains** White Rice Wheat Flour Corn
Starchy Vegetables Acorn Squash Yams Jicama Butternut Squash Gold Potatoes Parsnips Red Potatoes Artichoke Sweet Potatoes Pumpkin Purple Potatoes White Potatoes	**Starchy Vegetables** White Potatoes may cause inflammation for those sensitive to nightshades.
Fats and Oils Almonds Avocado Oil Almond Butter Cashews Almond Oil Cashew Butter Olive Oil Hazelnuts WalnutsChia Seeds Walnut Oil Sesame Seed Oil Hemp seeds Flax Seeds Avocado Brazil Nuts Pumpkin Seeds Pecans Macadamia Nuts Olives Sunflower Seed Butter	**Fats and Oils** Vegetable Oil Safflower Oil Soybean Oil Grape seed Oil Peanut Butter Mayonnaise Corn Oil
Herbs and Spices Turmeric Garlic Ginger Cinnamon Basil Thyme Black Pepper Sage Cilantro Parsley	Cayenne Pepper and Chili Pepper may cause inflammation to those sensitive to nightshades.

Cayenne Pepper Oregano Dill Mint Cloves Cumin	
Beverages Water Tea-Green, Black, White, Herbal, and Oolong	**Beverages** All other beverages should be avoided.
Nightshade Substitutions White Potato- Sweet Potato, Parsnips, or Turnips. Tomatoes- Beets, Pumpkin or Butternut Squash. Bell Peppers- Carrots, Celery, Cucumbers, or Radishes. Chili and Cayenne Pepper- Turmeric, Black Pepper, Cloves, Ginger or Garlic Powder. Eggplant- Portobello Mushrooms, Zucchini, or Okra.	

CHAPTER 8:

Foods Allowed and Foods to Avoid

Your diet can significantly impact your immune system. The microbiome (bacteria and microorganisms) in your digestive tract help to regulate your body's natural defense system. Everything you choose to eat will either cause inflammation or reduce it.

Choosing to consume a diet that consists of balanced fatty acids will help stifle low-grade chronic inflammation and enable you to feel your best. An essential anti-inflammatory diet focuses on removing sugary, processed foods, and adding fresh produce, healthy fats, whole, unprocessed grains, spices, and herbs. It is also vital to limit carbohydrates as they cause a significant amount of inflammation, as well.

Colorful vegetables are known to be a good source of antioxidants. Adding a great array of colorful vegetables and eliminating the starchy ones will help support your immune system.

Legumes are another great source of antioxidants and protein. To cut down on additives, try choosing dried beans and just soak they overnight before rinsing and cooking.

Grains can help reduce inflammation by supplying fiber and antioxidants if you choose the correct ones. Many people are sensitive to gluten, even those who do not have celiac disease; this can cause digestive and systemic inflammation. Be sure to choose gluten-free unprocessed grains such as whole oats, quinoa, barley, and brown rice.

Extra Virgin Olive Oil is high healthy fat and should be your go-to when cooking a meal or dressing a salad. Extra Virgin Olive Oil supplies monounsaturated fat, which can be useful for your heart and antioxidants, and a compound called oleocanthal, is known to lower inflammation.

While many foods should be included in your diet to reduce chronic inflammation, there are also some foods that you must avoid to help keep the swelling down.

Processed foods and sugars are two of the biggest culprits when it comes to inflammation in the western diet. Processed foods are highly refined, causing them to lose much of their natural fiber and nutrients. They are often high in omega 6, Tran's fats, and saturated fats, increasing inflammation.

Sugar is one of the worst offenders when it comes to increased inflammation. Not only does it hide in many foods, but studies have also found that it is very addictive. Because of this, you should expect to go through a withdrawal phase when you remove it from your diet. This can often cause headaches, cravings, and sluggishness. Give yourself some time to allow your body to work through it. Sugar, even natural sugars such as honey and agave, cause the body to release cytokines, which creates an immune response leading to inflammation. You don't have to remove natural sugars from your diet entirely, but you should only eat them a few times a week and at no more than one meal per day.

Most **fried foods**, especially deep-fried foods, should be avoided as well. Usually, they are cooked in processed oils or lard and are coated in refined flour that promotes inflammation. You will want to pay attention to foods known as nightshades. **Nightshades** can be anti-inflammatory, but some people are sensitive to them. If you find you seem to have more inflammation after consuming nightshade, you may want to begin making substitutions in your recipes. Below are many foods to increase in your diet and the ones you should limit or avoid. This list is not all-inclusive, so remember to stick to the above points.

CHAPTER 9:

How to Build a Diet That Works

A diet is a controlled and regulated regiment of food and drinks consumption designed to achieve a certain level of healthy living, induce weight loss, or reverse a pre-existing medical condition. Building a diet that works to its desired standard is not a comfortable fit; neither is it impossible. Dieting is an exercise that, when undertaken, would need to follow several cardinal rules, depending on the desired outcome of it all. A couple of these rules are below.

1. Identify and set goals for the diet.

Dieting is a deliberate effort to achieve a better life, health-wise. When one decides to go on a diet, they should have a mental picture of what they hope to gain from it. Whether it is weight loss, medical, or a test of the soul, there should be a list of what one aims to achieve. A timeline should guide goals set by a person, say daily, weekly, or monthly. The time-space could be in whatever form a person desires. If one feels that the goals set might be too hard to achieve, they should set milestones short-term wins. Generally, the mind is more receptive to an activity when there are wins and rewards involved.

2. Research on different types of diets and dietary needs.

When designing a regime to be followed during one's diet, it is vital to do extensive research on different available diets worldwide. If one is looking to borrow a diet sample from the internet, they should base their analysis on Body Mass Index, BMI, age, medical conditions, and fitness levels. These are but a few of the considerations that are made when researching. One should also consider their allergies and avoid foods containing such allergens, no matter how much such food may be hyped on the internet.

3. Make a diet that balances all classes of foods.

Balancing of foods is everything when it comes to dieting. All classes of foods, carbohydrates, protein, vitamins, and salts need to be considered equally and given priority in the diet. It is a common misconception that a diet comprised of protein and vitamins is more effective at weight loss. While it might accelerate fat burning, it deprives the body of carbs, which are the energy sources of the body, making it weak. A diet is just but a change in the intake of foods. It substitutes unhealthy foods for healthier eating. What it does not do is limit the consumption of a specific class of foods. That would be selective starvation.

4. Divide the meals into portions for consumption

Typically, people focus on three main meals of the day. However, most physicians and dieticians recommend that people should consume small portions several times a day. Several small portions allow the body to have a constant intake of nutrients throughout the day. They also prevent the alimentary canal from being overspent during the ingestion and digestion of food substances. Nutritionists recommend chewing one's food as much as possible to aid in easier digestion and reduce the rate at which fat builds up in the human body. Fast eaters are definitely at a loss over here.

5. Order meals in a timely fashion and consume all meals wholesomely.

All meals are essential for a healthier life. Skipping either one reduces the effectiveness of one's diet. Anorexic tendencies are highly discouraged. Remember, dieting is not about skipping meals or eating less food. Breakfast should be served at least 4 hours before the meal; be it lunch or a snack. Healthy snacks should be consumed in controlled amounts in between meals. Such snacks are in the classes of fruits, protein bars, and nutritional shakes. It is also essential to drink water in appropriate amounts, but the timing should be just right. Before and after meals, at least thirty minutes should pass for effective absorption into the bloodstream.

6. Work out alongside dieting.

Dieting alone could spur the aims that one hopes to achieve. Although this could work, it would significantly boost a diet's health benefits when regular exercise is introduced in the regime. Exercise regiments do not have to be intensive weight lifting and six-hour gym sessions. Exercise could be in the form of cardio, bodyweight training, also called calisthenics) or any other movement that is not normal to the body. Physicians all around the world recommend at least 30 minutes of exercise per day for a healthy life. Sweating it out has more benefits than the surface level tiredness it causes.

It opens up the skin pores and expels dirt from it while also targeting fat built up around muscles in the body.

7. Count daily calorie intake from foods

Calories are typically the energy building blocks of the systems combinations that make up the human body. However, in excess amounts, calories are what make people unhealthy and fat. Counting calories is one way to reduce the adverse effects of food on the human body. Doctors recommend that for a functional life, one should consume at least 1000 calories per day. The number of calories per serving should be counted according to the descriptions on the packaging. It would also help to search on the internet for the calorie specifications of different foods.

To sum up, it is essential to the points noted above. Dieting should be an undertaking that one views as a pleasure rather than a chore. Also, it helps to eat produce straight from the farm and cut down on processed foods. When the mindset is focused on change, and the will for betterment is present, a diet does more than inducing physical health. It will also spur mental, psychological, and emotional health. Finally, consistency and discipline are crucial when going on a diet. There is no pain without gain, and this is necessary when preceding pleasure foods for more healthy choices.

CHAPTER 10:

Sirtfood Diet Phases

Sirtfood diet emerged after an in-depth research on sirtuins was conducted which discovered seven proteins in the body that had the ability to enhance body metabolism, increase lifespan and reduce inflammation. The natural plant compounds discussed in the latter topic are responsible for activating the 'sirtuin gene' which leads to significant weight loss. The creators of the diet before making it happen, looked into all the available sirtfoods and chose the most effective foods in this category. The list of sirtfoods have been outlined in the prior topic.

To bring this into perspective, the originators of the diet came up with two phases that must be followed strictly to achieve the desired goal. The phases are broken down into phase 1 and 2, where each phase has its instructions. How you manage the two phases determine how the eventual result will look like. Some people do the two phases once, while others do them repeatedly until they each that fat-loss goal. Some of the sirtfoods in the diet are not very pleasant, it therefore calls for discipline and commitment in following the diet fully.

Sirtfood Diet Follows To Main Phases, Phase 1 And 2.

Phase 1 of the Sirtfood Diet

The first phase lasts for seven days. The first three days demand that you take three sirtfood juices combined with a full meal rich in sirtfoods. Here you can try one of the recipes provided. This comes to a total of 1,000 calories. In the next four days, the calorie intake can be increased to 1,500 by taking two sirtfood juices and two full meals on a daily basis. Two squares of dark chocolate are also included in this first phase of the diet.

In this first phase, it is advised that you should not take any alcoholic drink. The only permissible drinks at this stage are clean drinking water, tea, coffee and green tea. The first phase is highly embedded on calorie restriction. That is why the total calorie intake should not exceed 2,500 calories.

Phase 2 of the Sirtfood Diet

The Second phase does not necessarily focus on calorie restriction, but more of enriching the body with necessary nutrients to keep it going. Every day of the first phase requires one to take three-rich meal sirt food meals and a glass of green juice. Sirtfood bite snacks are allowed in this phase. Different from phase 1, red wine is allowed I n this phase, but must be taken in moderation. 2-3 glasses are allowed per week. The individual should not exceed this limit. Also, water, coffee and green tea are permissible. Phase 2 is referred to as the 14-day maintenance phase. Once this phase is over, sirtifying of other diets becomes the norm in order to achieve the weight loss goals.

For a positive response, one can repeat the two phases as many times and also for an effective fat-loss boost. Management of the two phases is quite important for one to achieve the objective of taking a sirtfood diet. Following every step of each step is essential as it allows the foods taken in to fulfill their role in the body of the user.

After one has fully completed the two phases effectively, it is good to sirtify I between meals. A point, one is allowed to take their favorite meal while giving it a sirtfood twist. However, one should be conscious of what they are taking, to avoid eroding the gains of the sirtfood diet. Foods taken after the two phases should be nutritious enough, in moderate quantities and prepared in a way that they maintain their nutritive value. The good thing is that we now have many recipes of sirtfood desserts, which one can choose from.

Managing phase 1 and 2 of a sirtfood diet

Phase 1 and 2 can be repeated as many times as possible for one to achieve that health boost and fat loss goal. Also, if you go off the track at some point, you can always go back and redo the phases.

Some of the participants that had been put under a sirtfood diet trial eventually showed that it is possible to lose a significant amount of Wight without much muscle loss. Majority of participants, especially who combined the diet with some form of exercises and gym, came out with well-toned bodies. An interview with one of the participant agreed that proper management of phase 1 and two is crucial to achieve good results. He reiterated that it demanded him a lot of displace, consistency and focus.

Following all the steps in Phase 1 and Two is not an easy task, it requires a lot of determination," one participant said.

The beauty of a sirtfood diet is that it works by burning fats hence weight loss. Furthermore, the diet promotes muscle growth, repair and maintenance. This is in contrast with other many available diets which have both loss of fats and muscle in order to lose weight. The flexibility of having a sirtfood diet is also on another level. Sirtfood diet can be incorporated with other meals and still achieve the desired result.

Once the individual has completed the diet following fully the two phases, it is encouraged that ne keeps including sirtfoods in their regular diets to prevent going back to the old unpleasant self. The signature sirtfood green juice is a must even after going through the phases. There are many Sirtfood Diet Books available, which have recipes that are easy to make. Majority of the sirtfood diet books have an elaborate explanation of how to follow Phase 1 and 2 in order to reach the main goal of weightless.

CHAPTER 11:

How to Lose Seven Pounds in Seven Days

Now that you have an idea of what a sirtfood diet is, it's time to start with stage one.

Below is the weekly plan you must follow as a starter. It could be shocking initially, especially if you came from a very unregulated diet, but this is the crucial point of any diet. If you can strictly follow this plan for the first week, you will form a good habit, and the following weeks will be easier for you, and the ensuing results will help you stay motivated. Don't be in a hurry, take your time, strictly follow the plan, and won't regret it.

Day1

Pick the juices at three distinct periods of the day, for example, as soon as you wake up, in mid-morning and in mid-afternoon, and select the regular or vegetarian dish.

You can use it as a reference to the recipes proposed.

Day 2

The second day, the formula is identical to that of the first one, and the only thing that changes is the substantial meal. Today you will also have dark chocolate and the same for tomorrow. This food is so fantastic that we don't need an excuse to eat it.

To earn the title of a "Sirt food," chocolate must be at least 85 percent cocoa. And even amid the various types of chocolate with this percentage, not all of them are the same.

Often chocolate is treated with an alkalizing agent to reduce its acidity and give it a darker color. Unfortunately, this process dramatically reduces the flavonoids activating sirtuins, compromising their benefits.

On day 2, capers take part in the menu. Despite what many may think, they are not fruits, but buds that grow in Mediterranean countries and are hand-picked.

They are perfect as Sirt foods because they are very rich in the nutrients kaempferol and quercetin.

For flavor, they are tiny concentrates of taste. If you've never used them, don't feel scared. They will taste astonishing if combined with the right ingredients; they will also give a unique and inimitable aroma to your dishes.

During the second day, you will intake three green Sirt juices and one substantial meal.

Drink the juices at three different times of the day, and choose either the normal or the vegetarian dish: for example Turkey escalope with capers, parsley, and sage on spiced cauliflower, couscous.

Day 3

You are now on the third day, and it's time to flavor everything with a fundamental ingredient.

For thousands of years, chili has been a milestone in the gastronomic experiences of the whole world.

As for the effects on health, we have already seen that its spiciness is perfect for activating sirtuins and stimulating the metabolism.

The applications of chili pepper are endless. You can use it everywhere; therefore, it's an easy way to consume Sirt food regularly.

If you are not an expert of chili, I recommend the Bird's Eye (Thai chili); it is the best for sirtuins.

The third day is the last you will consume three green juices daily; tomorrow, you will switch to two.

Take this opportunity to browse other drinks that you can consume during the diet. We all know that green tea is good for health, and water is naturally perfect, but what about coffee?

More than half of people drink at least one coffee a day, but always with a trace of guilt because some people say that it is an unhealthy habit, is untrue; studies show that coffee is a real treasure full of beneficial sub-stances.

That's why coffee drinkers run the least risk of getting diabetes, certain forms of cancer, and neurodegenerative diseases. Furthermore, not only is coffee, not a toxin, it protects the liver and makes it even healthier!

On the third day, you will intake three green Sirt juices and one substantial meal, regular or vegetarian.

Drink the juices at three different times of the day. Choose the regular or vegetarian dish: aromatic chicken breast with kale, red onion, tomato sauce, and chili or baked tofu with harissa on spiced cauliflower, for example.

Day 4

The fourth day of the Sirtfood Diet means that you are middle way through your journey to a thinner and improved body.

The significant change from the three days is that you will only drink two juices instead of three and that you will have two solid meals instead of one.

It means that on the fourth day and the upcoming, you will have two green juices and two solid meals.

The inclusion of Medjoul dates in a list of foods that promote weight loss and good health may seem shocking, particularly when you think they contain 66 percent sugar,

That has no stimulating properties towards sirtuins.

Conversely, it has well-known links with obesity, heart disease, and diabetes, just at the antipodes of the objectives, we aim to.

But industrially refined and processed sugar is very different from the sugar present in a portion of food containing sirtuin-activating polyphenols: the Medjoul dates. Unlike normal sugar, these dates, consumed in moderation, do not increase the glucose level in the blood.

Today we will also integrate chicory into meals. Like with onion, red chicory is better in this case too, but endive, its close relative, is also a Sirt food. If you are looking for ideas on using these salads, combine them with other varieties and season them with olive oil: they will give a spicy flavor to milder leaves.

On the fourth day, you will intake two green Sirt juices and

Two solid meals.

Drink the juices at different times of the day. Choose the regular or vegetarian dishes: muesli Sirt pan-fried salmon fillet with caramelized chicory, rocket salad, and celery leaves or muesli Sirt and Tuscan stewed beans.

Day 5

You have got the fifth day; now you can add fruits to your diet.

Due to its high sugar content, fruits have been the subject of bad advertising, except berries and Strawberries. They have shallow sugar content: one teaspoon per 100 grams. They also have an excellent effect on how the body processes simple sugars.

Scientists have found that if we add strawberries to simple sugars, this causes a drop in insulin demand, and therefore transforms food into a machine that releases energy for a long time. Strawberries are a perfect element in diets that will help you lose weight and get back in shape.

They are also delicious and extremely versatile, as you will discover in the Sirt version of the fresh and light Middle Eastern tabbouleh.

On the fifth day, you will eat two green Sirt juices and two solid meals.

As usual, Drink the juices at different times of the day, and choose between your regular or vegetarian dishes.

Day 6

Among the better Sirt foods, we have olive oil and red wine. Virgin olive oil is obtained from the fruit only by mechanical means, in conditions that do not deteriorate its propriety. You can be sure of its quality and polyphenol content. "Extra virgin" oil is that of the first pressing, "virgin" is the result of the second, and therefore has more flavor and better quality: this is what we suggest you use when cooking.

No Sirt menu would be complete without red wine, one of the keystones of the diet.

It contains the activators of resveratrol and piceatannol sirtuins, which probably explain the longevity and skinniness associated with the traditional French way of life, and which are at the origin of the enthusiasm unleashed by Sirt foods.

Wine contains alcohol, so, should be consumed with moderation. Pinot Noir is many people's favorite grape variety because it contains much more resveratrol than most of the others.

On the sixth day, you will assume two green Sirt juices and two solid meals

Drink the fluids at different times of the day, and choose the usual or vegetarian dishes: Super Sirt salad and grilled beef, fillet with red wine, onion rings, and roasted potatoes with aromatic herbs or lentil Sirt salad and mole sauce of red beans with roasted potato.

Day 7

The seventh day is the last of stage one of the diet.

Considering it as a beginning, because you are about to embark on a new life, in which Sirt foods will play an essential role in your nutrition.

Sunday's menu is a perfect example of how easy it is to integrate abundance into your daily diet. Just take your favorite dishes, and, with a touch of creativity, you will turn them into a Sirt meal.

Walnuts are excellent Sirt food, unlike current opinions. They have high-fat content and many calories, yet it has been shown that they reduce weight and metabolic diseases due to the activation of sirtuins. They are also a multipurpose ingredient, excellent in baked dishes, in salads and as a snack, alone.

Pesto is becoming an exceptional ingredient in the kitchen because it is tasty and allows you to give character to even the simplest dishes.

The traditional recipe is made with basil and pine nuts, but you can try an alternative with parsley and walnuts. The result is delicious and rich in Sirt foods.

We can apply the same idea to an easy-to-prepare dish, such as an omelet. The dish must be the typical recipe appreciated by the whole family, and simple to transform into a Sirt dish with a few little tricks.

In our recipe, we use bacon. It fits perfectly. The Sirtfood Diet tells us what to include, not what to exclude, and this allows us to change our long-term eating habits. After all, isn't that the secret to not getting back the lost pounds and staying healthy?

On the seventh day, you will assume two green Sirt juices and two solid meals.

Drink the juices at different times of the day and choose the usual or vegetarian dishes: Sirt omelet Sirt and baked aubergine wedges with walnut and parsley pesto and tomato salad.

CHAPTER 12:

Sirtfood with Other Food

We traveled deeper and deeper into Sirtfood' beautiful universe, we started to understand how big their application could be. We are well aware that no two people eat the same. Many health-conscious individuals are firmly dedicated to eating, with the likes of paleo, low-carbon, intermittent fasting, and gluten-free diets becoming especially common. Although for others they aren't effective, some swear by them.

But how will these blend into Sirtfood?

A lightbulb moment struck with the understanding that if Sirtfood were introduced into them, any of those typical diets would be significantly enhanced. The advantages people obtained from the health or weight loss can be increased in adequate amounts by adding Sirtfood. Sirtfood are similar in respect: if there is a way to eat that does well for you, adding Sirtfood into it will make the results much better.

We're both busy physicians, so our passion for Sirtfood has evolved. We've steadily incorporated Sirtfood into the clients' diets, irrespective of their favorite eating process. Our inference is clear: Sirtfoods is consistent with all other nutritional strategies, but they are also effectively enhancing. Indeed in any healthy diet, they should be important ingredients. Overlook them, and you lose a trick.

Low-Carb Diet

Low-carb diets have been a significant trend on the weight-loss map ever since Atkins, the founder of low-carb diets, rose to meteoric prominence. Subsequent reincarnations have tended to power the low-carb trend, such as the Dukan diet. Between them, they have notched up to tens of millions in diet- sales. While these low-carb diets can be severe, especially in their early phases of "attack," their strong feelings reflect a broader change in opinion towards an anti-sugar and even anti-carbon stance. Citizens are gradually fleeing the sinking ship of the low-fat ideology, and the changing loyalties towards the "carbs are the enemy" camp.

One of the Sirtfood Diet's uniqueness is that it doesn't include this territorial dispute. It's an inclusive diet, which ensures you don't have to pick sides to remove a whole range of foods from your lifestyle to reach the body you desire. Nonetheless, we know that many people choose a lower-carb eating style, so where does Sirtfoods come in?

If you are encouraged to be low-carb, we advise you not to scrimp on Sirtfoods, but to accept them. Some of the main pitfalls we find in people slipping into when eating low-carb diets in our professional practice is the shortage of plant-based ingredients that they provide. Meals are primarily focused around meat (most sometimes refined beef), fish, milk, cheese, and other dairy products, and vegetable-based diets are confined to the bottom of the pecking order. Yet if its low carb, we're told it's all fine, or so.

Sadly, faced with nearly everything we know about nutrition and health, the belief that plant-based foods are not vital in our diets flies. A diet stripped from the overwhelming amount of healthy compounds present in plant foods can do nothing to avert an explosion of infectious disorders such as diabetes, heart disease, and cancer. And the surplus of Sirtfoods can easily be blended into a carb-restricted way of eating. Only look at the top twenty Sirtfoods list, and you'll figure that a huge majority of them are relatively weak in carbohydrates. We are talking of an abundance of leafy and low-carb vegetables (arugula, celery, endive, cabbage, and onions), culinary herbs (garlic, parsley), spices (chili, turmeric), capers, walnuts, chocolate, and extra virgin olive oil, not to mention the drinks (coffee and green tea). As for fruit, too much the focus of targeting low-carb diets, even the strawberries weigh in a generous 31/2-ounce (100 g) portion with a pure teaspoon of carbohydrates.

The bottom line for us is this: a low-carb diet would not be a low-Sirtfood diet. Incorporating Sirtfoods not only improves a low-carb diet's weight-loss advantages but also significantly raises its health potential.

Intermittent Fasting/the 5:2 Diet
Over the past few years, intermittent fasting, also known as IF, has become a major culinary trend, epitomized by the 5:2 diets' runaway popularity. That usually includes restricting calorie consumption on two days a week to between 500 and 600 calories a day and consuming whatever you want on the other five days.

While solid work on the effects of intermittent fasting is minimal, it does seem to be helpful for weight loss and boost some of the disease risk factors. But as we have shown, it is not appropriate for large portions of the population, it induces unnecessary loss of muscle, and it is only successful if you can stick to it. And that's always the elephant in the house when it comes to extended fasting and why we don't enjoy it so much. In our clinical context, for some considerable amount of time, most individuals refuse to adhere to intermittent fasting regimens. Hunger is an uncomfortable sensation that is gnawing away at you, and naturally, people don't like getting hungry.

Although intermittent fasting hasn't turned out to be a panacea, it's famous for a cause, and fans would swear by its advantages. Of course, we appreciate this. But why not make a significant improvement to your fast by "Sirtifying" it?

With the addition of Sirtfoods, you will get all the advantages they offer, from helping to satiate hunger and conserve muscle, to reduce the negative effects of fasting. But their presence has yet another major bonus. You'll note that fasting's benefits are induced by triggering our sirtuin genes, which is also exactly how Sirtfoods function. That means you can boost your calorie intake to a far more achievable amount while still reaping all the same benefits with Sirtfoods now present to share the fasting "burden."

That is exactly what we find in our clinical experience. Followers have been able to raise their energy consumption from the last 500 to 600 calories on quick days to a far more achievable 800 to 1,000 calories with only the addition of Sirtfood-rich green juices (the same recipe included in this) into a regular IF diet.

And if your penchant is for extended fasting, by not accepting Sirtfoods, you're losing a trick and making short days unduly grueling. There's also a whole new perspective from which intermittent fasting diets will

Benefit from accepting Sirtfoods.
There is very little, if any, emphasis on the consistency of the food for IF diets; it's just about the calorie loss on the fast days. The proponents are vociferous in supporting the notion that on non-fast days you should eat whatever you want. It doesn't even seem to care if what you eat is good, mediocre, or awful. Yet, as we know, to keep anything running in tip-top condition, the body requires a constant supply of vital nutrients. Can we

hope to remove the body of essential calories by eating whatever nutrient-stripped, refined foods we choose, mainly though we fast for two days and stay away from chronic diseases such as Alzheimer's or heart disease?

What if, on the other hand, nutrient-dense Sirtfoods were also used on your non-fasting days? You will undoubtedly be eating fat and just two days a week enhancing your health — it will be seven today. To us, this development of the sporadic approach to fasting is a no-brainer. It's the equivalent to replacing a full-color HD black-and-white Set.

Paleo Diet

In a nutshell, the paleo diet advocates that before the introduction of western agriculture and more recently industrial food production, we would consume the diets that our ancestors were meant to consume. Essentially we're talking of a diet-style hunter-gatherer or caveman consisting of meats, seafood, shellfish, vegetables, fruits, and nuts, while banished to the forest are dairy foods, cereal grains, starch, and other refined food.

They raise this question for paleo dieters: what could be more paleo than consuming the plant foods we have coevolved that turn on our ancient sirtuin genes? You must note that both plants and animals have evolved ways to deal with frequent environmental pressures such as drought, exposure to the sun, lack of nutrients, and aggressor attacks. Plants have evolved particularly sophisticated stress-response mechanisms because of their sedentary nature (they can't run away!), creating a complex assortment of polyphenols that allow them to cope with their environment. For decades, these polyphenols have been eaten by humans, piggybacking on these sophisticated plant-produced stress-response signals and reaping huge benefits as they turn to our sirtuin genes.

How might we more paleo than drinking the plant-activating sirtuin compounds on which our hunter-gatherer forebears thrived? The missing piece of paleo theory is sirtfood.

Gluten-Free Diet

For those wanting to stop gluten, the advantage of the Sirtfood Diet is that the top twenty Sirtfoods are all naturally gluten-free. Gluten is a protein that is present in maize, rye, and barley.

Many individuals with a gluten allergy (through cross-contamination) may also be prone to oats. The autoimmune celiac disorder, affecting as much as 1 in 100 people in America, is hypersensitive to gluten and cannot be ingested in some way. Yet, apart from this very severe gluten allergy, several citizens are progressively experiencing gluten-free.

Diets and sometimes they have a great outlook on them.

As people embark on gluten-free diets, which include taking out staples like bread, pasta, and the myriad of other foods made from gluten-containing grains, one of the major issues is that the diet is nutritionally deficient and no longer offers the full variety of nutrients and fibers needed to stay in good health. What's so amazing about the Sirtfood Diet is that one of our top Sirtfoods is buckwheat, a naturally gluten-free and highly nutritious pseudo-grain, which, as we've seen in the s, is flexible enough to serve as a substitute for gluten-containing grains, whether in the form of flour, pasta, flakes or noodles (check the box carefully to make sure they are 100 percent).

The better diets are, of course, the ones that are complex and interesting, not bland and monotonous. We also have shown that quinoa, another pseudo-grain, is not just gluten-free, it often has substantial quantities of sirtuin-activating nutrients, rendering it the great buckwheat replacement. Aside from its normal appearance as a plant, quinoa is widely available from natural food retailers and online niche vendors in rice, chips, and pasta.

With quinoa and buckwheat taking center stage, it's happier days for those following a gluten-free diet: they provide a healthy alternative to certain grains and bring some strong Sirtfood credentials to the regular diet as staple products.

We cannot end the issue of gluten-free diets without a word of advice about the amount of gluten-laden processed food that is now filled in the supermarket's "free-from" shelves. They are the finely processed, dried, sugar-free, gluten-free alternatives to pies, pancakes, cookies, cereals for breakfast, etc. That has become a big industry, but please do not slip into the pit of believing that it is inherently safe only because a food is gluten-free. Most of these foods are junk nutritionally pure, just like their counterparts, which contain gluten. If you are adopting a gluten-free diet, we advise you to take your health and well-being to a whole new stage with a diet rich in naturally gluten-free syrtle foods, not gluten-free garbage.

What food can't you consume with a sirtfood diet?

Officially, there is no food you can't consume on the Sirtfood Diet, but the calorie restriction is severe, especially within the first three days you're restricted to 1,000 calories.

CHAPTER 13:

Why You Need to Follow the Sirtfood Diet

It is proven that the Sirte diet makes you lose at least three kilos in a week because, by activating the sit-ins, it allows you to burn fat faster. Since it is not a question of excluding foods but of supplementing them, this diet is also easy and pleasant to follow and has numerous advantages. For example, it does not upset habits; it is compatible with all food regimes, it does not force prohibitive renunciations, it does not make the lean mass lose weight, that is, the muscles but only the fat, it does not regain the lost pounds, it does not make you feel hungry, does not ruin social life, helps to keep cholesterol and blood sugar under control and is also approved by many doctors and nutritionists.

In addition to the foods listed above, here are other foods that contain substances that can activate sit-ins in abundance: extra virgin olive oil, buckwheat, red wine, walnuts, soy, caper, cocoa, parsley, coffee, celery, cabbage, red radicchio, rocket, red onion, and dates.

Example of Sirt food Diet Menu
Breakfast: juice with Sirte food, then, for example, strawberry or apple and a blueberry smoothie (blueberries are another food rich in sit-ins

Snack: three walnuts and an apple

Lunch: pasta with cabbage pesto

Snack: fruit salad of strawberries and blueberries

Dinner: steamed fish with vegetable garnish

Sirte diet: minus 3.5 kg in a week

1. **Small goals, long-lasting results**

Too many drastic changes to one's diet do not go far. It is better to set more limited objectives, but more specific and more comfortable to achieve. Starting from a change - in a healthy key - in quality, the difference in quantities will also come. Some examples: substitute sauces and dips with extra virgin olive oil and spices; choose a whole meal for bread, pasta, and cereals.

- ## Calories and portions, no calculator needed

We now know (almost) everything about the properties of foods, thanks to more and more numerous articles and TV programs on the subject. Deciding without guilt is not difficult, even if you are queuing at the bar under the office, and your minutes are counted. Greenlight for large portions for those dishes rich in water and vegetables such as soups, velvets, salads, and - the fashion of the moment - Hawaiian pokes. On the contrary, limit the consumption of bread or croutons served in the accompanying bowl. If you fancy a carbonara, eat it without pairing it with other caloric dishes like eggplant parmigiana or a slice of cake. The same goes for pizza but giving up on frying.

1. ## Beware of sugar

Muffins, cheesecakes, cupcakes, cream biscuits, donuts, multilayer cakes, pastries ... They are colorful, Instagram able, and immediately bring joy, but they are also rich in sugars. Limit the consumption of pastry products; you will gain in health, and the scale will thank you. Then there are the "hidden" sugars, such as those contained in ketchup, in sauces for seasoning salads, and in canned products: the important thing is not to consume them habitually.

1. ## Mindfulness also at the table.

Weight control is not just a matter of numbers and sizes. The awareness is crucial when it comes to power because what we eat provides us with the necessary energy for work and leisure, or - if we too often bad choices - heavy and extra pounds. Taken from the commitments of everyday life, we often do not even remember what we ate for breakfast. Savoring every bite of your meal - and understanding when you are exaggerating with quantities - is instead a gesture of love for yourself. Do not order the first thing that happens: make a correct choice, carve out a moment of gratitude for the food you are eating and ask yourself why you have opted for one dish instead of another.

1. **X-ray snacks**

Munching one snack after another while at the desk or in front of the TV is the easiest way to store unnecessary and harmful sugars and fats. Before grabbing yet another snack, listen to your appetite and ask yourself: "Am I starving? Do I need it? ". Say no to junk food to calm anger, and negative thoughts: better chew chewing gum or drink something, breathe deeply, and eat something healthier after a few minutes. Some suggestions: Greek yogurt sweetened with honey instead of the usual pudding; almonds and peanuts natural (in modest quantities) instead of the salty or sugary versions; rice chips and legumes or Grana Padano, cooked in the oven, instead of the classic chips; natural berries in place of candied fruit; vegetables in pinioned instead of fries.

6) **Planned transgressions**

Weight control should not turn into a constant source of anxiety. Take pen and paper or, if you are more used to technology, download one of the many dedicated apps, and draw up a calendar of transgressions. Choose a day - better yet, two half days - where you can eat what you prefer and enjoy your favorite foods as if you tasted them for the first time. You will appreciate them even more. Some additional attention is required in the ceremonial season. If you take part in two or more weddings in a month, those will be the days of transgression, and there will be no others.

7) **Aperitifs, Netflix ... A reality check is needed**

The food calendar will help you take into account other risk factors for your silhouette. If the aperitifs with friends and colleagues multiply during the summer, make an effort not always to eat the same things at every happy hour. If you love binge-watching on Netflix, schedule a healthy snack every two episodes. Are you afraid of an upcoming visit to the dentist? Opt for an herbal tea, a, or a relaxing massage instead of muffins and fries.

- **Chew slowly**

Even if you have a thousand job commitments or are absorbed in a river conversation with your BFF, try to chew slowly. Your digestive tract will thank you. It takes between 15 and 20 minutes for the body to digest and absorbs nutrients, sending a satiety signal to the mind. By chewing slowly, you will be able to recognize that signal, avoiding ingesting unnecessary calories.

9) Plan with drinks

Don't focus your dietary efforts only on snacks. Some cocktails, such as mojito and piña colada, are a real bomb of sugar and calories and could frustrate your efforts. Attention also to industrial fruit juices. In the first case, a glass of wine or a small mug of beer is preferable. In the second, a freshly prepared smoothie.

1. **Protein, live balance**

Excessive consumption of animal meat and protein is harmful to health (and the environment). You don't have to become vegan; you just have to alternate between animal and vegetable protein consumption. Foods such as legumes, cabbage, and spinach are essential sources of energy and, thanks to fiber's contribution, a valid aid for intestinal regularity

CHAPTER 14:

How to Follow the Sirtfood Diet to Achieve Your Weight Loss Goals

One step at a time! That's what it takes to incorporate sirtfood into your diet. The diet is simple and easy to follow in a sense that it only calls for a few definite steps to take. Firstly, you will need to increase food consumption that is rich in sirtuin, then you will have to follow the phases of the diet plus you will need to add green juices to your daily diet. Here are a couple of steps that must be followed to achieve your weight loss goals on a sirtfood diet:

Get the right ingredients.
Remember that all this diet asks from you is to increase your sirtuins intake. That can be done only through careful and selective grocery shopping. Prepare a list of the ingredients that contain a high amount of sirtuins and check their utility as per your meal plan. There are certain ingredients like coffee, parsley, red wine, and chocolate that you can have all the time. So, stock up your kitchen cabinets with these ingredients.

Set up the schedule
The sirtfood diet gives you small weight loss targets for each week. In the initial period, you must prepare a schedule to keep track of your meals, the caloric intake, and the timing of green juices you are consuming in a day. In this way, you will be able to easily manage the first few days of the diet adoption and continue observing body changes and measuring your weight to keep track of your pace.

Prepare for the first week.
In the first week of the sirtfood diet, the dieter must control his caloric intake. Therefore, to avoid any mistakes or confusion, all the high caloric food items should be removed from sight. Stuff your refrigerator only with the food appropriate for the sirtfood diet, and keep the juices, fruits, and vegetables ready to use. Instead of planning your meal every other day, make plans for the entire week according to the caloric limitations.

Prepare your meals

Now that you have read the list of Sirt foods, it's time to plan your menu to shop for all your required ingredients. If possible, aim to buy your fresh ingredients every few days and include Sirt foods in every meal.

By far, the best way to load up on those Sirt foods is to start your day with a healthy smoothie. Especially a green one as it's a great refreshing kick start to your body, and you can easily pack in 5 fruits/vegetables in one drink. It's sure to keep hunger away too!

If you have had a busy day and haven't been able to pack in the Sirt goodies as much as you would like, you can always supplement with a handful of walnuts, a green tea or a coffee in between meals to give you a boost and keep hunger away.

If you are careful with your calorie intake, you can be guided by the information on each recipe. A little word of caution when it comes to dates or 'nature's toffees' as some people call them – they are rich in calories. One date contains around 61 calories, so don't go overboard. That said, if you would typically reach for cakes, sweets, or biscuits then a date or two is a good substitute because you will not be consuming empty refined sugar calories, yet still enjoying a sweet treat.

Caloric intake

Keep in mind that sirtfood is more about weight loss, so mere sirtuins cannot magically work overnight if you keep consuming more calories than your body can burn. Do the math and understand your caloric needs, even when the diet does not restrict you from high caloric intake after the first seven days. You must maintain a strict check on the daily caloric intake to keep the weight in control. Otherwise, it does not take much to regain the lost pounds.

Green juices

Green juices are one of the essential parts of the sirtfood diet. These are your way to detoxification and quick weight loss. Green veggies are full of phytonutrients, minerals, and antioxidants. Having them frequently throughout the day can help boost the metabolism, remove the metabolic waste from the body, and enables the body to metabolize the needed nutrients appropriately. These juices are also great for keeping electrolyte balance in the body.

Maintenance

To harness the benefit of this diet or any other diet, it is imperative to maintain your new dietary routine. Most people abandon the diet as soon as they are an oven with the first two phases of the diet or achieve their weight loss goals. Soon, they regain weight and blame the diet for being ineffective, far from reality. It all depends on how consistently you follow this diet plan.

Conclusion

The Sirtfood diet was created by two nourishment specialists that, as of late, co-composed about the diet. Before you run out and get it, how about we set aside you some cash and give you the down and out here.

The part that interests sound eaters and dieters is that these proteins seem to confine calories, or impact our digestion, a reaction of which is known to slow maturing in numerous species.

Sirtuins strengthen the immune system, help build muscle, and ensure that cell metabolism decreases - in other words, the aging process is slowed down, you stay "young longer". All you need to do is switch to foods that activate many sirtuins.

A preliminary of the diet among exercise center goers demonstrated fast weight loss, yet the centers for the most part around smart dieting – which we at HelloFresh love!

The step is to test out all of the recipes and follow along with each of the phases with the proper foods and drinks. Follow the two planned stages, Phase 1 and Phase 2, and you will be guaranteed to enjoy more energy, vitality, a lighter feeling, and on average, about 7 lbs. Lighter on the scale each week.

Though a relatively new diet, it is proven to be effective and yields fast and safe results. As a bonus, you can still eat chocolate and enjoy drinking wine!

In addition to the aesthetic changes that you will see, it is actually what is "inside" those counts. Achieving optimum health is now possible with the numerous health benefits of the Sirtfood diet. I promise you that the quality of your life will undoubtedly be improved; all it takes is adding those healthy sirtuin-rich foods!

Also, this diet is prescribed to drink up to three glasses of juice per day. Although this juice can be a good source of vitamins and minerals, it contains almost no healthy fiber needed by the body. Also, the diet is so limited in calories and food choices that it is highly likely to lead to a deficiency of protein, vitamins, and minerals, especially at the first stage.

Due to its low-calorie content and limited choice of food, this diet can be challenging to follow for all three weeks. Adding here the high costs of buying a juicer, , and some rare and expensive ingredients, as well as spending time preparing unique dishes and juice, the diet becomes completely unfeasible for many people.

Health is wealth, they say. Eating the right foods as well as maintaining the right lifestyle will not only help you to keep fat away but will also help to keep sicknesses and diseases away.

The Sirtfood diet has several benefits that you will enjoy. This has brought together to Understand what is Sirtfood Diet how to Begin to ensure that you get the complete nutrition that your body needs. It will help you to understand the process of the Sirtfood Diet Plan. Start to Boost your Energy and Activate your Metabolism for a Healthy Lifestyle. this will guide you on how to start your proper Sirtfood Diet Meal Plan. Variety of good recipes that will guide you to achieve your ideal weight goal without Starving.

I hope this guide has helped you become acquainted with the Sirtfood diet and achieve your weight loss and health goals. Good luck on your sirtfood journey!

Bibliography

Article title: The Sirtfood Diet: A Detailed Beginner's Guide

Website ti-tle: Healthline

URL: https://www.healthline.com/nutrition/sirtfood-die

Article title: Our Core Science - Why Sirtuins Are Important | Elysium Health

Website ti-tle: Elysium Health

URL: https://www.elysiumhealth.com/en-us/science-101/why-sirtuins-are-important-for-aging

SIRTFOOD DIET COOKBOOK:

SECRET RECIPES TO ACTIVATE METABOLISM, BURN FAT, BOOST YOUR ENERGY AND EAT HEALTHIER. A HEALTHY DIET PLAN FOR A FAST WEIGHT LOSS AND TO LEARN A HEALTHIER LIFESTYLE.

MEGAN LEAN

TABLE OF CONTENTS

Introduction:

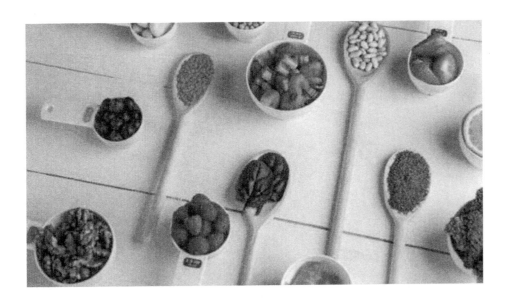

The Sirtfood Diet

Sirtfood Diet was developed in the United Kingdom by two nutritionists who were working at a private gym. They marketed the diet as a "revolutionary new diet" and health strategy that works by switching on the "skinny gene" in the human body system.

The Sirtfood diet is the latest way to burn extreme body fat and loses weight dramatically without having to experience malnutrition or starve oneself. Activating the skinny gene is achieved through exercising and fasting. There are some categories of foods that have chemicals known as polyphenols that when consumed, they put little stress on the body cells. Thus, producing genes that imitate the consequences of both fasting and exercise. Certain foods have high polyphenols present in them, such as dark chocolate (cocoa), coffee, red wine, kale, and so on. When these kinds of foods are taken, they tend to release Sirtuins reactions that influence aging, mood, and metabolism. Any diet high in Sirtfoods triggers weight loss without necessarily having to expend muscles, while at the same time maintaining a healthy lifestyle and health.

This diet focuses on calorie restriction, which is in phases. This calorie restriction is believed to increase the production of Sirtuins in the body.

Is Sirtfood Diet Good for You?

Every food on the diet plan is extremely healthy for you. You stand to get the right amount of nutrients, vitamins, and minerals, which will likely become high when following this diet. This diet is very restrictive on some kinds of foods and calories, and this may make it a bit difficult for some people to follow and get accustomed to.

Sirtfood Diet Essentials

The diet consists of twenty highly rated foods, which you can combine with your everyday meal.

I. **Buckwheat**:- This is available in the form of noodles and fruit seed. It's in every way different from wheat. So, when getting yours, it should be 100 percent buckwheat.

II. **Celery** -Very nutritious, especially the hearts and the leaves. Always blend hem.

III. **Extra virgin olive oil**: -This is a very top ingredient in SIRTFOOD DIET. It has a peppery taste, and it's highly sirtifying.

IV. **Bird's eye chilli** -Also known as Thai chili. They are hotter than regular chili's and have more nutrients.

V. **Capers** - Good for salad.

VI. **Green tea or matcha** - Very soothing when combined with a slice of lemon.

VII. **Cocoa** - Helps in the control of blood sugar, cholesterol, and blood pressure.

VIII. **Kale** - It's a very high SIRTUINS activator. Rich in quercetin and kaempferol.

IX. **Parsley** - Sprinkle it on your meals, juice, or smoothies. It's far more than just a mere garnish.

X. **Lovage** - Best known as a digestive Aid

XI. **Red onion** – Know to have Antibacterial Properties

XII. **Strawberries** - Antioxidants

XIII. **Chicory** – Use to lose of Appetite, Upset Stomach, Constipation

XIV. **Turmeric** – Helps Prevent Cancer and Boost Immune System

XV. **Soy** – High Source of Omega-3 Fatty Acid
XVI. **Red wine** – Healthy heart and Antioxidant
XVII. **Walnuts** – Decrease Inflammation, Rich in Antioxidants
XVII. **Medjool dates** – Good Source of Fibers
XIV. **Rocket** – Calcium, Vitamin C, Vitamin K

Does Sirtfood Diet Have Any Side Effects?

First and foremost, the diet has no room for substitutions. Sirtfood Diet is very limiting and restrictive. It counts calories and focuses on a specific food category. Even though the SIRTFOOD recommended meals may look yummy and tasty, the diet is likely to be deficient in significant nutrients like iron, zinc, and calcium. They are not the kind of meal you will most likely find on the "list of healthy food," says an anonymous nutritionist. Eating a little bar of chocolate and having a glass of red wine is no bad thing and won't affect the body in any way. However, it shouldn't be an everyday thing. Eating varieties of fruits and vegetables is better and not just the ones recommended on the list.

Also, the weight loss can only be maintained only if the calorie restriction is also maintained; otherwise, the weight comes right back. It takes time to burn fat and loses weight; there's no doubt about this. This kind of weight loss is most likely to be that of fluid and not fat. The moment people go back to their former lifestyle and eating habit, the weight will be back in a matter of time, except if this is long term diet.

If you are not the type that skips food regularly, especially during the day, you are very much likely to experience some difficulties such as dizziness, headaches, nausea, and inability to concentrate.

CHAPTER 1:

How to Activate Your "Skinny Gene" Without Fasting

There are 2 phases of the Sirtfood diet. The first, which lasts one week, is meant to activate your "skinny gene" and the following 2 weeks are intended to maintain your Sirtuins level up and ensuring an overall better metabolism. After that, you will have to maintain a healthy and sirtfood rich diet

But let's start with the first seven days. You will find handy meal plans for the early seven days

Phase 1: 7 pounds in 7 days

The phase 1 of the Sirtfood diet is the one that will allow you to take the first successful step towards achieving a leaner shape and a healthier glow.

The authors of the diet proved with their clinical trial that no matter your initial weight or gender, you will lose 7 pounds in 7 days, and it won't be muscle mass!

This is not the most amazing part of the diet, the fact that the lost pounds won't come back to haunt you is! After all, the first week of the diet is based on the simple, well-proven base of calorie restriction, but with the added twist of a sirtfood-laden meal plan.

Not only will you see an improvement of your shape, but you will feel more vital, your skin will achieve a natural glow that no cream can ever compete with. I was skeptical at first, too, but I never felt so energetic, clean, and beautiful.

Phase 1 of the diet is the one that produces the greatest results. Over seven days, you will follow a simple method to lose 3.5 kg.

During the first three days, the intake of calories will have to be limited to one thousand per day at most. You can have three green juices and a substantial meal, all based on Sirt foods. From day 4 to 7, the daily calories will become fifteen hundred. Every day you will eat two green juices and two solid Sirt-meals. By the end of the seven days, you should have lost, on average, 3.5 kilos.

Despite the reduction in calories, the participants do not feel hungry, and the calorie limit is an indication rather than a goal. Even in the most intensive phase, calorie restriction is not as drastic as in many other regimes. Sirtfoods have a naturally satiating effect so that many of you will feel pleasantly full and satisfied.

Phase 1 plan:

Days 1 to 3 – max. 1000 calories

3 green juices

1 main Sirtfood meal

Think of these first 3 days as the reset button for your metabolism. I swear it isn't as grueling as it seems. The match in the green juice and the SIRT-activating of the foods will satisfy and make you feel more energetic than ever.

Day's 4 to 7 – max. 1500 calories

2 Green juices

2 main Sirtfood meals

You can choose amongst different types of juicers, depending on your needs and financial possibilities. Let's take a look at the choices:

Centrifugal juicers:

Centrifugal juicers do just that; they use centrifugal force to spin the food (most like vegetables like carrots, cucumbers, or kale leaves) at high speeds to the sidewalls, where there are blades. The food is pushed through a sieve, and then you have your juice. You have to drink this rather quickly, as you will lose nutrients the longer it is exposed to air (which it already has done as it was spinning), and it oxidizes, as well as a bit of heat from the friction which creates a loss of nutrients and enzymes. This is the whole reason you are juicing, so this point is quite important. You are also left with a lot of solid but very wet pulp as a byproduct, which also means there were a lot of fibrous parts of the plants that the juicer couldn't handle. This is also a missed opportunity for more nutrients. You will also get a lot of (warmish) foam at the top, which some people do not like. It is quick, and it is easy, however, and it is usually the cheapest of the juicer types. If you must, it is better than not having one at all, but if you can invest, you will reap your rewards.

Masticating juicers:

Masticating juicers also do what they say they are. They masticate or chew the food, albeit more slowly than the other type, by pulling it through gears that extract the juice. The machine pushes the pulp out. You would have less pulp with this machine afterward. There is also less oxidation, and thus, more nutrients. They also can handle other types of foods (which vary by make and model), but that is something you should consider. You will get some foam with this as well, but not as much. These are more expensive, and again, should be looked at as you would an investment that you would not use and toss away. If you want it to last, and you want to get the most from your juicing and take it seriously, you will want to spend a bit more money and get what you need.

Triturating juicers:

These geared juicers have geared that grind together with millimeters of space left between, to tear open foods, and grind the plants with only a dehydrated pulp that is left. These are the most nutrient-efficient juicers on the market. They leave virtually no foam, and they are nutrient-dense as they are not disturbing the inner plant cells with oxidation. You usually can tell in the look (color) and taste (more luxurious) than other juices. You can use different attachments to make different foods with most brands as well, so they are versatile. These are the highest pricing of most of the juicers in general, and there are also brand variations as with the others.

Stock your fridge and pantry

First, clear your cabinets and refrigerator of foods that are unhealthy, and that might tempt you. You also will have a very low-calorie intake at the start, and you do not want to be tempted into a quick fix that may set you back. Even though you will have new recipes, you may feel that your old comfort foods are more natural now.

Then, go shopping for all the ingredients that you will need for the week. If you buy what you will need, it is more cost-effective. Also, once you see the recipes, you will notice that many ingredients overlap. You will get to know your portions as you proceed with the diet, but at least you will have what you need and save yourself some trips to the store.

Wash, dry, cut, and store all the foods that you need that way; you have them conveniently prepared when you need them. This will make a new diet seem less tedious.

Prepare in advance

The lack of time often thwarts a resolution for a change in diet. So, knowing this, prepare. You can easily prepare the meals the night before to take to work the day after instead of getting tempted by a cafeteria sandwich. Juices can be prepared in bulk and stored. They will keep in the fridge for 3 days and even longer in the freezer. You must protect them from light and add the matcha only when you are ready to consume them.

Get used to eating early

Drink your juices as the earlier meals in the day if it helps you. It is a great way to start your day for three reasons: (1) it will give you energy for breakfast and lunch especially. By not having to digest heavy foods, your body saves time and energy usually spent on moving things around to go through all the difficult motions. You will be guaranteed to feel lighter and more energetic this way. You can always change this pattern after the maintenance phase, but you may find that you want to keep that schedule. (2) Having fruits and vegetables before starchy or cooked meals, no matter how healthy the ingredients are the best way to go for your digestion. Fruits and vegetables digest more rapidly, and the breakdown into the compounds that we can use more readily. Think of it as having your salad before your dinner. It works in the same way. The heavier foods, grains, oils, meats, etc., take more time to digest. If you eat these first, they will slow things down, and that is where you have a backup of food needing to be broken down. This is also when you may find yourself with indigestion. (3) Juices, especially green juices, contain phytochemicals that not only serve as antioxidants, but they contribute to our energy and mood. You will notice that you feel much differently after drinking a green juice than you would if you had eggs and sausage. You may want to make a food diary and note things such as this!

be mindful of what you are drinking

Besides the mandatory green juices, you should feel free to drink freely: plain water, black coffee, and green tea are recommended. Do not drink soft drinks and fruit juices! To make your water tastier and more "SIRT-full," you can add some sliced strawberries to cold sparkling water.

Eat until you are 80% full

It's an Okinawan proverb, and it couldn't be truer. Sirtfoods will more than satisfy your appetite; you might even find yourself feeling full before finishing your meal, don't force it down!

Think of the journey and not the destination

This is not a diet to lose weight; it's a change in lifestyle and a celebration of the most diverse culinary traditions. Take joy in cooking and knowing that you are eating well. Focus on the path rather than the destination, and you will find it much easier to follow the diet.

Phase 2: 14 days of Sirtfoods

Phase 2 is the maintenance phase and lasts 14 days. During this period, although the main objective is not the reduction of calories, you will consolidate weight loss and continue to lose weight.

The secret to succeeding at this stage lies in continuing to eat Sirtfoods in abundance: during these two weeks, you will consume three balanced and abundant Sirtfoods per day and a green SIRT-juice.

This part of the diet plan is a lot more of a healthy eating plan than a 'diet plan' per se. Besides the 3 healthy Sirtfood meals a day, you are permitted plus 1 or 2 little treats. Drinks-wise you are still limited to green tea, coffee, black tea, and water. However, you are now allowed to have 2-3 glasses of red wine per week

This diet is unlike other diets where it does not end; it truly becomes a part of your lifestyle and could be a permanent way of eating. There would be no restrictions after the traditional diet has ended. When you get past Phase 2, you can eat from Sirtfoods as you please. The other great thing about Sirtfood food is that you can go back to Phases 1 and 2 at any time. You have the tools, and you will have the recipes. You will also feel more confident about creating your recipes using a variety of Sirtfoods.

The best part about the Sirtfood diet is that anyone can enjoy the juices, smoothies, cooked meals, or desserts. They are not restrictive, and you can eat them and get creative with Sirtfood ingredients for the rest of your long and healthy life.

CHAPTER 2:

Grocery Shopping List for the Sirtfood Diet

Dark Chocolate

A great source of flavanoids, dark chocolate (the kind that's at least 70% cocoa and unprocessed), can improve your health in a number of ways. A small piece of dark Chocolate is a great cure for your sugar cravings and it boosts your endorphins and serotonin levels at the same time. The chemicals found in Chocolate can also help fight stroke, heart disease, and high body pressure.

Red Wine

Red wine has antioxidant, anti-inflammatory properties and even cancer-fighting potentially. Made from purple grape skins and seeds, This beverage is high in polyphenols and Resveratrol, which can help protect blood vessels from damage, reduce bad cholesterol, and prevent blood clots. Stick to one glass a day to reap the benefits.

Onions

Red onions are not only a low-calorie, flavor-boosting addition to any meal, they may also reduce your risk of developing certain cancer, due to the compounds qQuercetin. Onions are a significant source of antioxidants and are rich in vitamin C which gives your immune system a welcomed boost.

Green Tea

Green tea is Made up of antioxidant that help protect our cells from damage and catechins which may play a role in increasing our metabolic rates. Look for matcha tea since its Made from crushed tea leaves themselves so it packs a more powerful punch.

Blueberries

Blueberries Have been found to help lower bad cholesterol, fight signs of aging, reduce inflammation in the body, and help you burn fat. Thanks to the high antioxidant count also as all the phytonutrients, This dark berry may be a snack you'll enjoy daily.

Coffee

Now you have more reason to enjoy your morning cup of coffee. Along with giving you an energy boost, it can also increase your endurance when exercising, reduce your risk of certain diseases, and potentially improve brain function.

Parsley

Extremely high in chlorophyll, which is a strong antioxidant. Parsley also has alpha-linolenic acids, which is an omega-3 that can fight heart disease and arthritis. The luteolin in This herb May also protect your eyes as well.

Turmeric

Another superfood, Turmeric is often used in ayurvedic treatments, thanks to it being antiseptic, anti-inflammatory, and rich in antioxidants. Curcumin, the compounds found in Turmeric, not only gives the Spice its beautiful bright color, but May also prevent Alzheimer's, certain cancers, and blood clots.

Olive Oil

Another ingredient that can lower bad cholesterol, Olive oil is full of monounsaturated fatty acids which can also help regulate insulin and blood sugar too. Stick to two tablespoons a day to get the antioxidant your body needs without overdoing it on the Calorie front.

Earth's - Eye Chili. Additionally, sold as Thai chilies, they truly are stronger than ordinary chilies and packed with more nutritional elements. Utilize them to increase sour or sweet recipes.

Buckwheat

Technically a pseudo-grain: it's a berry seed linked to rhubarb. Additionally, accessible noodle shape (like soba), but ensure that you're getting the wheat-free edition.

Capers.

If you are wondering, then they are pickled flower buds. Sprinkle them a salad or roasted steaks.

Celery.

The leaves and hearts would be the most healthful part, and thus do not throw them off if you are mixing a shakeup.

Chicory.

Red is most beneficial, but yellowish works too. Include it into a salad.

Cocoa.

The flavonol-rich type enhances blood pressure, blood glucose cholesterol, and control. Search to get a high proportion of cacao.

Extra Virgin Steak Oil.
The extra-virgin type includes more Sirt benefits, and a far more pleasing, flavor.

Green Tea or Matcha.
 Add a piece of lemon juice to raise the absorption of sirtuin-producing nutritional elements. Matcha is much better, but go Japanese, not Chinese, to steer clear of potential lead contamination.

Kale.
Includes huge levels of sirtuin-activating nutrition quercetin and kaempferol. Scrub it with coconut oil and lemon juice serves it as a salad.

Lovage.
It is an herb. Grow your personal onto a windowsill and throw it into stirfries.

Medjool Dates
They truly are a hefty 66 percent glucose, however in moderation -- do not raise glucose levels, also have been connected to reduced levels of diabetes and cardiovascular disease.

CHAPTER 3:

Sirtfood Diet Breakfast

1. Cranberry Quinoa Breakfast

Preparation Time: 10 Minutes

Cooking time: 20 minutes
Servings: 2
Ingredients:
½ cup quinoa
1 cup milk
2-3 tbsp. honey, optional
1 tsp cinnamon
½ tsp vanilla
1 tsp ground flaxseed
2 tbsp. walnuts or almonds, chopped
2 tbsp. dried cranberries
Directions:
Rinse quinoa and drain.
Combine milk, quinoa, and flaxseed into a saucepan.
Bring to a boil, add in cinnamon and vanilla and simmer for about 15 minutes.
When done, place a portion of the quinoa into a bowl, drizzle with honey, and top with cranberries and crushed walnuts.
Nutrition:
Calories, 48g
Carb, 9g
Fat, 1g Sat.
Fat, 8g
Fiber.5g

2. Green Omelet

Preparation Time: 10 minutes
Cooking time: 30 minutes
Servings: 2
Ingredients:
2 large eggs, at room temperature
1 shallot, peeled and chopped
Handful arugula
3 sprigs of parsley, chopped
1 tsp extra virgin olive oil
Salt and black pepper
Directions:
Beat the eggs in a small bowl and set aside.
Sauté the shallot for 5 minutes with a bit of the oil on low-medium heat.
Pour the eggs in the pans, stirring the mixture for just a second.
The eggs on medium heat and tip the pan just enough to let the loose egg run underneath after about one minute on the burner.
Add the greens, herbs, and the seasonings to the top side as it is still soft.
Tip: you do not even have to flip it, as you can just cook the egg slowly egg as is well (being careful as not to burn).
Tip: Another option is to put it into an oven to broil for 3-5 minutes (checking to make sure it is only until it is golden but burned).
Nutrition:
Calories: 296.

Sodium: 557 mg.

Fat: 19g.

Fiber: 2 g.

Protein: 25 g

3. Berry Oat Breakfast Cobbler

Preparation Time: 10 minutes
Cooking time: 40 minutes
Servings: 2
Ingredients:
2 cups of oats/flakes that is ready without cooking
1 cup of blackcurrants without the stems
1 tsp of honey (or ¼ tsp of raw sugar)
½ cup of water (add by testing the pan)
1 cup of plain yogurt (or soy or coconut)
Directions:
Boil the berries, honey, and water and then turn it down on low.
Put in a glass container in a refrigerator until it is cool and set (about 30 minutes or more)
When ready to eat, scoop the berries on top of the oats and yogurt.
Serve immediately.
Nutrition:
Calories: 344
Carbohydrates: 50g
Fat: 15g
Protein10g
Fiber10g
Sodium: 18mg
Cholesterol: 1mg

4. Pancakes with Apples and Blackcurrants

Preparation Time: 10 minutes
Cooking time: 20 minutes
Servings
Ingredients:
2 apples cut into small chunks
2 cups of quick-cooking oats
1 cup flour of your choice
1 tsp baking powder
2 tbsp. raw sugar, coconut sugar, or 2 tbsp. honey that is warm and easy to distribute
2 egg whites - 1 ¼ cups of milk (or soy/rice/coconut)
2 tsp extra virgin olive oil - A dash of salt
For the berry topping:
1 cup blackcurrants, washed and stalks removed
3 tbsp. Water (may use less)
2 tbsp. Sugar (see above for types)
Directions:
Place the ingredients for the topping in a small pot simmer, frequently stirring for about 10 minutes until it cooks down, and the juices are released.
Take the dry ingredients and mix them in a bowl.
After, add the apples and the milk a bit at a time (you may not use it all), until it is a batter.
Stiffly whisk the egg whites and then gently mix them into the pancake batter.
Set aside in the refrigerator.
Pour a one-quarter of the oil onto a flat pan or flat griddle, and when hot, pour some of the batters into it in a pancake shape.
When the pancakes start to have golden brown edges and form air bubbles, they may be ready to be gently flipped.
Test to be sure the bottom can change life away from the pan before flipping.
Repeat for the next three pancakes.
Top each pancake with the berries.
Nutrition:
Calories: 120.8 Dietary Fiber: 3.1 g Carbohydrate: 18.7 g Total Fat: 1.2 g

5. Sweet and Savory Guacamole

Preparation Time: 10 minutes
Cooking time: 20 minutes
Servings: 2
Ingredients:
2 large avocados, pitted and scooped
2 Medjool dates, pitted and chopped into small pieces
½ cup cherry tomatoes cut into halves
5 sprigs of parsley, chopped
¼ cup of arugula, chopped
5 sticks of celery, washed, cut into sticks for dipping
Juice from ¼ limes
Dash of sea salt
 Directions:
Mash the avocado in a bowl, sprinkle salt, and squeeze of the lime juice.
Fold in the tomatoes, dates, herbs, and greens.
Scoop with celery sticks and enjoy!
Nutrition:
Calories: 156
Fiber: 1.3g
Carbohydrates: 1.4g
Protein 3.4g
Fat: 15.2g

6. Buckwheat Pita Bread

Preparation Time: 10 minutes
Cooking time: 20 minutes
Servings: 2
Ingredients:
1 tbsp. Packet dried yeast

2 tbsp. Polenta for dusting

3 tbsp. of olive oil

2 cups lukewarm water

2 cups buckwheat flour

1 tsp of sea salt
Directions:
Combine the yeast and water and let the mixture activate (approximately 10 to 15 minutes).
Combine the buckwheat flour, olive oil, salt, and add in the yeast mixture.
Knead it slowly until you make the dough.
Cover and place in a warm spot for about an hour (to rising).
Evenly divide the dough into six pieces.
Take a piece, shape it to a flat disc, and then place it in between 2 sheets of baking paper.
Carefully roll out the dough into ¼-inch thick round pita shapes.
Using a fork, pierce the dough a couple of times and lightly dust it with the polenta.
Heat a 10-inch cast-iron and smear it with olive oil.
Cook the bread on one side until puffy then do the same with the other side.
Fill up with desired vegetables and meat and serve immediately.
Alternatively, you could wrap it in foil, place it in the fridge, and reheat in the oven the next day.
Nutrition:
Total Fat: 100
Carbohydrate: 20g
Fat: 0g
Protein: 3g

7. Smoked Salmon Omelet

Preparation Time: 10 minutes
Cooking time: 10 minutes
 Servings: 2
Ingredients:
1 tsp. Chopped Rocket

Smoked Salmon, Sliced

1 tsp of extra virgin olive oil
½ tsp of capers
2 medium eggs
1 tsp of chopped parsley
Directions:
Crack the eggs into a bowl and whisk them well.
Add the capers, parsley, rocket, and salmon and heat oil in a non-stick pan until hot but not smoking.
Add the egg mixture into the pan and move it around the pan using a spatula.
Reduce the heat to low and let the omelet cook.
Slide the spatula under the omelet, fold it up in half, and serve.
Nutrition:
Total Fat: 303
Carbohydrate: 1g
Fat: 22g
Protein: 23g

8. Breakfast Scramble

Preparation Time: 10 minutes
Cooking time: 20 minutes
Servings: 2
Ingredients:
A handful of button mushrooms, sliced thinly
1 tsp of mild curry powder
½ tsp. of parsley, chopped finely
½ bird's eye chili, sliced thinly
1 tsp of ground turmeric
2 eggs
1 tsp of extra virgin olive oil
1 tsp. kale, chopped roughly
Optional-add seed mixture as toppings and rooster sauce for flavor
Directions:
Mix the curry powder and turmeric, and then add a little water until you have a light paste.
Steam the kale for about 2 to 3 minutes.
Place a frying pan over medium heat and heat the oil.
Fry the mushroom and chili for 2 to 3 minutes until they start to soften and brown.
Add the paste, cook the eggs, and then serve.
Nutrition:
Total Fat: 261
Carbohydrate: 10g
Fat: 19g
Protein: 13g

9. Strawberry Buckwheat Tabbouleh

Preparation Time: 10 minutes
Cooking time: 20 minutes
Servings: 2
Ingredients:
4 tbsp. of tomato
1 tbsp. of ground turmeric
3 tbsp. Buckwheat

1 tbsp. Extra Virgin Olive

2 tbsp. Parsley

2 tbsp. Hulled Strawberries

2 tbsp. Rocket

4 cups Avocado

1 tbsp. Red Onions

1 tbsp.. Capers

Half Lemon Juice

2 tbsp. Medjool Dates Pitte

Directions:
Cook the buckwheat and the turmeric following the packet directions
Drain, and then set aside to let it cool.
Finely chop the avocado, parsley, red onion, tomato, dates, and capers and mix it with the cool buckwheat.
Slice strawberries and gently mix into the salad together with the lemon juice and oil.
Serve them on a bed of rocket.
Nutrition:
Total Fat: 208
Carbohydrate: 16g
Fat: 11g
Protein: 7g

10. Easy Quinoa Crackers

Preparation Time: 10 minutes
Cooking time: 40 minutes
Servings: 2
Ingredients:
2 cups cooked quinoa
1 cup ground flaxseed
2 tbsp. sesame seeds
1 tbsp. honey
1 tsp salt
1 cup of water
3 tbsp. extra virgin olive oil
1 tsp garlic powder (optional)
½ tsp dried oregano (optional)
Directions:
Thoroughly mix all ingredients in a large bowl.
Place the dough on a lined baking sheet and, with wet hands, flatten the dough.
Slip the parchment off the baking sheet, cover the length of the dough with plastic wrap and roll out the dough with a rolling pin to a ¼ inch thickness.
Bake at 350 f for 35 minutes or until the parchment paper quickly pulls away, and the dough is cooked but not crisp yet.
Flip the cracker over, gently remove the parchment paper and cut into squares.
Bake for another 35 minutes, or until the crackers are nice and crisp.
Nutrition:
Total Fat: 150
Carbohydrate: 12g
Fat: 10g
Protein: 5g

11.   Granola-The Sirt Way

Preparation Time: 10 minutes
Cooking time: 50 minutes
Servings: 2
Ingredients:
1 cup buckwheat puffs
1 cup buckwheat flakes (ready to eat type, but not whole buckwheat that needs to be cooked)
½ cup coconut flakes
½ cup Medjool dates, without pits, chopped into smaller, bite-sized pieces
1 cup of cacao nibs or very dark chocolate chips
½ cup walnuts, chopped
1 cup strawberries chopped and without stems
1 cup plain Greek, coconut, or soy yogurt.
Directions:
Mix, without yogurt and strawberry toppings.
You can store it for up to a week. Store in an airtight container.
Add toppings (even different berries or different yogurt).
You can even use the berry toppings as you will learn how to make from other recipes.
Nutrition:
Total Fat: 210
Carbohydrate: 32g
Fat: 5g
Protein: 10g

12.   Ginger Prawn Stir-Fry

Preparation Time: 10 minutes
Cooking time: 40 minutes
Servings: 2
Ingredients:
6 prawns or shrimp (peeled and deveined)
½ package of buckwheat noodles (
5-6 leaves of kale, chopped
1 cup of green beans, chopped
5g Lovage or celery leaves
1 garlic clove, finely chopped
1 bird's eye chili, finely chopped
1 tsp fresh ginger, finely chopped
2 stalks celery, chopped
½ small red onion, chopped
1 cup chicken stock (or vegetable if you prefer)
2 tbsp. Soy sauce
2 tbsp. extra virgin olive oil
Directions:
Cook prawns in a bit of the oil and soy sauce until done and set aside (about 10-15 minutes).
Boil the noodles according to the directions (usually 6-8 minutes).
Set aside.
Sauté the vegetables, then add the garlic, ginger, red onion, chili in a bit of oil until tender and crunchy, but not mushy.
Add the prawns, and noodles, and simmer low about 5-10 minutes past that point.
Nutrition:
Total Fat: 294
Carbohydrate: 22g
Fat: 12g
Protein: 25g

13.   Chicken with Mole Salad

Preparation Time: 10 minutes
Cooking time: 35 minutes
Servings: 2
 Ingredients:
1 skinned chicken breast
2 cups spinach, washed, dried and torn in halves
2 celery stalks, chopped or sliced thinly
½ cup arugula
½ small red onion, diced
2 Medjool pitted dates, chopped
15 ml. of dark chocolate powder
15 ml. extra virgin olive oil
30 ml. Water
5 sprigs of parsley, chopped
Dash of salt
Directions:
In a food processor, blend the dates, chocolate powder, oil and water, and salt.
Add the chili and process further.
Rub this paste onto the chicken breast and set it aside in the refrigerator.
Prepare other salad mixings, the vegetables, and herbs in a bowl and toss.
Cook the chicken in a dash of oil in a pan, until done, about 10-15 minutes over a medium burner.
When done, let cool and lay over the salad bed and serve.
Nutrition:
Total Fat: 289
Carbohydrate: 28g
Fat: 9g
Protein:28g

CHAPTER 4:

Sirtfood Diet Lunch Recipes

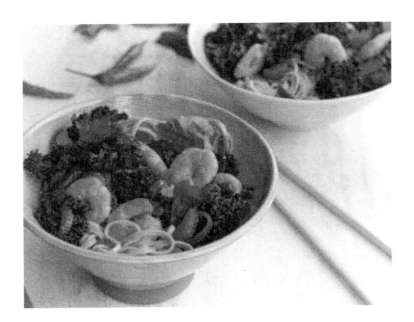

14.   Sticky Chicken Watermelon Noodle Salad

Preparation Time: 20 minutes
Cooking time: 40 minutes
Servings: 2
Ingredients
2 pieces of skinny rice noodles
1/2 tbsp. sesame oil
2 cups watermelon
Head of bib lettuce
Half of a lot of scallions
Half of a lot of fresh cilantro
2 skinless, boneless chicken breasts

1/2 tbsp. Chinese five-spice
1 tbsp. extra virgin olive oil
Two tbsp. sweet skillet (I utilized a mixture of maple syrup using a dash of tabasco)
1 tbsp. sesame seeds
A couple of cashews - smashed
Dressing - could be made daily or 2 until
1 tbsp. low-salt soy sauce - 1 teaspoon sesame oil
1 tbsp. peanut butter - Half of a refreshing red chili
Half of a couple of chives
Half of a couple of cilantros
1 lime - juiced
1 small spoonful of garlic

Directions:

In a bowl, then completely substituting the noodles in boiling drinking water. They are going to be soon spread out in 2 minutes.

On a big sheet of parchment paper, throw the chicken with pepper, salt, and the five-spice.

Twist over the paper subsequently flattens the chicken using a rolling pin.

Place into the large skillet with 1 tbsp. of olive oil, turning 3 or 4 minutes, until well charred and cooked through.

Drain the noodles and toss with 1 tbsp. of sesame oil onto a sizable serving dish.

Place 50% the noodles into the moderate skillet, frequently stirring until crispy and nice.

Remove the watermelon skin, then slice the flesh to inconsistent balls, and then move to plate.

Wash the lettuces and cut into small wedges and half of a whole lot of leafy greens and scatter on the dish.

Place another 1 / 2 the cilantro pack, the soy sauce, coriander, chives, peanut butter, a dab of water, 1 teaspoon of sesame oil, and the lime juice in a bowl, then mix till smooth.

set the chicken back to heat, garnish with all the sweet sauce (or my walnut syrup mixture) and toss with the sesame seeds.

Pour the dressing on the salad toss gently with clean fingers until well coated, then add crispy noodles and then smashed cashews.

Mix chicken pieces and add them to the salad.

Nutrition:

Calories: 694 Carbohydrates: 0 Fat: 33g Protein: 0

15.   Fruity Curry Chicken Salad

Preparation Time: 20 minutes
Cooking time: 10 minutes
Servings: 2
Ingredients
 Original recipe yields 8 servings
Fixing checklist
4 skinless, boneless chicken pliers - cooked and diced
 1 tsp celery, diced
 4 green onions, sliced
 1 golden delicious apple peeled, cored, and diced
 1/3 cup golden raisins
 1/3 cup seedless green grapes, halved
 1/2 cup sliced toasted pecans
 ⅛ Teaspoon ground black pepper
 1/2 tsp curry powder
 3/4 cup light mayonnaise
Directions:
In a big bowl, combine the chicken, onion, celery, apple, celery, celery, pecans, pepper, curry powder, and carrot. Mix altogether. Enjoy!
Nutrition:
Fat; 44 milligrams

Cholesterol: 188 milligrams

Sodium. 12.3 g

Carbohydrates: 15.1 gram of

Protein; full nutrition

16.   Zuppa Toscana

Preparation Time: 25 minutes
Cooking time: 60 minutes
Servings: 2
Ingredients
  1 lb. ground Italian sausage
  1 1/4 tsp crushed red pepper flakes
  4 pieces bacon, cut into ½ inch bits
  1 big onion, diced
  1 tbsp. minced garlic
  5 (13.75 oz.) can chicken broth
  6 celery, thinly chopped
  1 cup thick cream
  1/4 bunch fresh spinach, tough stems removed
Directions:
Cook that the Italian sausage and red pepper flakes in a pot on medium-high heat until crumbly, browned, with no longer pink, 10 to 15minutes. Drain and put aside.

Cook the bacon at the exact Dutch oven over moderate heat until crispy, about 10 minutes. Drain, leaving a couple of tablespoons of drippings together with all the bacon at the bottom of the toaster. Stir in the garlic and onions cook until onions are tender and translucent, about five minutes.

 Pour the chicken broth to the pot with the onion and bacon mix; contribute to a boil on high temperature. Add the berries and boil until fork-tender, about 20 minutes. Reduce heat to moderate and stir in the cream and the cooked sausage – heat throughout. Mix the lettuce to the soup before serving.
Nutrition:
Carbohydrates; 32.6 g

Fat; 45.8 g

Carbs; 19.8 g

Protein; 99 Milligrams

Cholesterol: 2386

17. Turmeric Chicken & Kale Salad with Honey-Lime Dressing

Preparation Time: 20 minutes
Cooking time: 10 minutes
Servings: 2
Ingredients
For your poultry
 1 tsp ghee or 1 tablespoon coconut oil
 1/2 moderate brown onion, diced
 250 300 grams / 9 oz. Chicken mince or pops upward chicken thighs
 1 large garlic clove, finely chopped
 1 tsp turmeric powder
 Optional 1teaspoon lime zest
 Juice of 1/2 lime
 1/2 tsp salt
For your salad
 6 broccoli 2 or two cups of broccoli florets
 2 tbsp. pumpkin seeds (pepitas)
 3 big kale leaves, stalks removed and sliced
 Optional 1/2 avocado, chopped
 Bunch of coriander leaves, chopped
 Couple of fresh parsley leaves, chopped
For your dressing
 3 tbsp. lime juice
 1 small garlic clove, finely diced or grated
 3 tbsp. extra virgin coconut oil (I used 1. tsp avocado oil and 2 tbsp. Eva)
 1 tsp raw honey
 1/2 tsp wholegrain or Dijon mustard
 1/2 tsp sea salt
Directions:
 Heat the ghee or coconut oil at a tiny skillet pan above medium-high heat. Bring the onion and then sauté on moderate heat for 45 minutes, until golden. Insert the chicken blossom and garlic and simmer for 2-3 minutes on medium-high heat, breaking it all out.
 Add the garlic, lime zest, lime juice, and salt and soda and cook often stirring to get a further 3-4 minutes. Place the cooked mince aside.

As the chicken is cooking, add a little spoonful of water. Insert the broccoli and cook 2 minutes. Rinse under warm water and then cut into 3-4 pieces each.

Insert the pumpkin seeds into the skillet out of the toast and chicken over moderate heat for two minutes, often stirring to avoid burning. Season with a little salt. Set-aside. Raw pumpkin seeds will also be nice to utilize.

Put chopped spinach at a salad bowl and then pours over the dressing table. With the hands, massage, and toss the carrot with the dressing table. This will dampen the lettuce, a lot like what citrus juice will not steak or fish Carpaccio– its "hamburgers" it marginally.

Finally, toss throughout the cooked chicken, broccoli, fresh herbs, pumpkin seeds, and avocado pieces.

Nutrition:
Calories: 266 Kcal
Protein: 99 milligrams
Carbohydrates: 0g

18. Buckwheat Noodles with Chicken Kale & Miso Dressing

Preparation Time: 15 minutes
Cooking time: 15 minutes
Servings: 2
Ingredients
For the noodles
2 3 handfuls of kale leaves (removed from the stem and fully trimmed)
150 g / 5 oz. buckwheat noodles (100 percent buckwheat, no wheat)
34 shiitake mushrooms, chopped
1 tsp coconut oil or ghee - 1 brown onion, finely diced
1 moderate free-range chicken, chopped or diced
1 red chili, thinly chopped (seeds out based on how hot you want it)
2 large garlic cloves, finely chopped
23 tbsp. tamari sauce (fermented soy sauce)
For your miso dressing - 1 ½ tbsp. fresh organic miso
1 tbsp. tamari sauce - 1 tbsp. peppermint oil
1 tbsp. lime or lemon juice - 1 tsp sesame oil (optional)

Directions:
Bring a medium saucepan of water. Insert the kale and cook 1 minute, until slightly wilted. Remove and put aside but keep the water and put it back to boil. Insert the soba noodles and cook according to the package directions (usually about five minutes). Rinse under warm water and place aside.

meanwhile, pan press the shiitake mushrooms at just an extraordinarily little ghee or coconut oil (about a tsp) for 23 minutes, until lightly browned on each side. Sprinkle with sea salt and then place aside.

in the exact skillet, warm olive oil ghee over medium-high heating system. Sauté onion and simmer for 2 3 minutes and add the chicken bits. Cook five minutes over medium heat, stirring a few days; you can put in the garlic, tamari sauce, and just a tiny dab of water. Cook for a further 2-3 minutes, often stirring until chicken is cooked through.

Last, add the carrot and soba noodles and chuck throughout the chicken to heat up.

Mix the miso dressing and scatter on the noodles before eating; in this manner, you can retain dozens of enzymes that are beneficial at the miso.

Nutrition:
Calories :694 Carbohydrates: 0g Fat: 33g Protein: 99 milligrams

19. Asian King Prawn Stir Fry Together with Buckwheat Noodles.

Preparation Time: 10 minutes
Cooking time: 10 minutes
Servings: 1
Ingredients:
shelled raw king prawns, deveined
Two tsp tamari (it is possible to utilize soy sauce if you aren't quitting gluten)
Two tsp extra virgin coconut oil
soba (buckwheat noodles)
1 garlic clove, finely chopped
1 bird's-eye chili, finely chopped
1 tsp finely chopped ginger
red onions, chopped
2 tbsp. celery, trimmed and chopped
6 tbsp. green beans, sliced
4 tbsp. kale, approximately sliced
1 tsp. Lovage or celery leaves
Directions:
Heating a skillet on high heat, cook the prawns into 1 tsp of this tamari and one tsp of the oil 2--three minutes. Transfer the prawns into your plate. Wipe out the pan with kitchen paper, even because you are going to make use of it.
Cook the noodles in boiling water --8 minutes as directed on the package. Drain and put aside.
Meanwhile, squeeze the garlic, chili and ginger, red onion, celery, lettuce, and beans at the rest of the oil over medium-high temperature for two-three minutes. Bring the stock and bring to the boil, then simmer for a moment or two, before the veggies have been cooked but still crunchy.
Insert both the prawns, noodles, and Lovage/celery leaves into the pan, then returns to the boil and then removes from heat and serve.
Nutrition:
Fat: 11.2g
Saturated: 1.6g
Carbohydrates: 70g

20.   Baked Salmon Salad with Creamy Mint Dressing

Preparation Time: 10 minutes
Cooking time: 20 minutes
Servings:
Ingredients
1 salmon shrimp (4oz.)
2 tbsp. mixed salad leaves
2 tbsp. young spinach leaves
2 radishes, trimmed and thinly chopped
5cm slice cucumber, cut into balls
2 spring onions, trimmed and chopped
1 small number parsley, roughly sliced
Dressing:
1 tsp low-fat mayonnaise
1 tbsp. organic yogurt
1 tbsp. rice vinegar
2 leaves mint, finely chopped
Salt and freshly ground black pepper
Directions:
Preheat the oven to 200°c (180°c fan/gas 6).
Get the salmon fillet onto a baking dish and bake for 16--18 minutes until cooked. Remove from the oven and place aside. The salmon is every bit as fine cold or hot in the salad. If your fish contains skin, then just brush down the skin and eliminate the salmon out of the skin using a fish piece after ingestion. It will slide easily once cooked.
In a small bowl, combine the mayonnaise, yogurt, rice vinegar, coriander leaves, and salt and salt and leave to stand for at least 5 minutes to permit the flavor to develop.
Arrange the salad lettuce and leaves onto the serving plate and top with the radishes, cucumber, spring onions, and parsley. Flake the carrot on the salad and drizzle the dressing.
Nutrition:
Calories: 340g
Carbs: 0
Cholesterol:0

CHAPTER 5:

Sirtfood Diet Dinner Recipes

21.   Bang-Bang Chicken Noodle Stir-Fry Recipe

Preparation Time: 10 minutes
Cooking time: 60 minutes
Servings: 2
Ingredients 1 tbsp. sunflower oil
package chicken thighs, boned, any surplus skin trimmed
1 cup frozen chopped mixed peppers
Inch courgette, peeled into ribbons, seeded center chopped
1 chicken stock cube - 1 cup. pack moderate egg yolks
4 garlic cloves, finely chopped
1/2 tsp crushed chilies, and additional to serve (optional)
4 tbsp. reduced-salt soy sauce - 2 tsp caster sugar
1 lime, zested, 1/2 juiced, 1/2 slice into wedges to function
Directions:
Heat the oil in a skillet on medium-low warmth. Fry the chicken skin-side down to 10 mins or until your skin is emptied. Flip and simmer for 10 mins, or until cooked. Transfer to a plate cover loosely with foil. Reheat the wok over a high temperature, add the peppers and sliced courgette; simmer for 5 mins. Meanwhile, bring a bowl of water to the boil, and then crumble in the stock block, adding the noodles. Simmer for 45 mins until cooked, and then drain well. Insert the garlic and crushed chilies into the wok; simmer for two mins, in a bowl mix the soy sugar and the lime juice and zest. Enhance the wok, bubble 2 mins; you can add the courgette noodles and ribbons. Toss with tongs to coat in the sauce. Cut the chicken into pieces. Divide the noodles between 4 bowls and top with the chicken. Serve with the lime wedges along with extra crushed chilies in case you prefer.
Nutrition: Calories: 718g Carbs: 0 Cholesterol: 0

22.   Cajun Steak and Veg Rice Jar Recipe

Preparation Time: 10 minutes
Cooking time: 20 minutes
Servings: 2
Ingredients
2 tbsp. vegetable oil
1 celery stick, finely chopped
3 large carrots, sliced into rounds
1 cup frozen chopped mixed peppers
4 spring onions, chopped, green and white parts split
2 cups 5 percent beef mince
2 teaspoon seasoning
1 teaspoon tomato purée
2 x 1 cup packs ready-cooked long-grain rice

Directions:
Heat the oil in a large, shallow skillet over moderate heat. Add the carrots, celery, peppers, and snowy areas of the nuts. Cook for 10 mins before the veg is beginning to soften.

Insert the mince, season liberally, and cook for 10 mins before mince is browned and start to go crispy.

Insert the Cajun seasoning and tomato purée; stir fry to coat the mince. Hint inside the rice combined with 4 tablespoons of plain water. Stir to unite heat and heat until the rice is hot ultimately. Scatter on the rest of the spring onion before serving.

Nutrition:
Calories: 518kcal
Carbohydrates: 4g
Protein: 34g
Fat: 39g
Cholesterol: 160mg
Sodium: 869mg
Potassium: 585mg

23.   Pesto Salmon Pasta Noodles

Preparation Time: 10 minutes
Cooking time: 30 minutes
Servings: 2
Ingredients
1.5 cup penne

2 x 1 cup tins cherry salmon, drained

1 lemon, zested and juiced

1 cup jar green pesto

1 cup package cherry tomatoes halved

8 tbsp. bunch spring onions, finely chopped

8 tbsp. package reduced-fat mozzarella

Directions:
Preheat the oven to windows 7, 220°c, buff 200°c. Boil the pasta for 5 mins. Drain, reserving 100ml drinking water.
Meanwhile, at a 2ltr ovenproof dish, then mix the salmon, lemon zest, and juice, then pesto (booking 2 tablespoons) berries and half of the spring onions; season.
Mix the pasta and reserved cooking water to the dish. Mix the allowed pesto using 1 tablespoon water and then drizzle on the pasta. Gently within the mozzarella, top with the rest of the spring onions and bake for 25 mins until golden.
Nutrition:
Calories: 407.75g
Total Fat: 9.2g
Cholesterol: 78.3g
Carbs: 44.9g

24.   Sri Lankan-Style Sweet Potato Curry

Preparation Time: 10 minutes
Cooking time: 40 minutes
Servings: 2
 Ingredients
1/2 onion, roughly sliced
3 garlic cloves, roughly sliced
2 tbsp. slice ginger, chopped and peeled
1 tbsp. fresh coriander, stalks and leaves split, leaves sliced
Two 1/2 tablespoon moderate tikka curry powder
4 tbsp. package cashew nuts
1 tbsp. olive oil
2 cups Red Mere farms sweet potatoes, peeled and cut into 3cm balls
2 cups tin isle sun coconut-milk
1/2 vegetable stock block
1 cup grower's harvest long-grain rice
1 cup frozen green beans
½ cup Red Mere farms lettuce
1 lemon, 1/2 juiced, 1/2 cut into wedges
To function
 Directions:
Set the onion, ginger, garlic, coriander stalks tikka powder along with half of the cashew nuts in a food processor. Insert 2 tablespoons water and blitz to a chunky paste.
At a large skillet, warm the oil over moderate heat. Insert the paste and cook, stirring for 5 mins. Bring the sweet potatoes, stir, and then pour into the coconut milk and stock. Bring to the simmer and boil for 25-35 mins before the sweet potatoes are tender.
Meanwhile, cook the rice pack directions. Toast the rest of the cashews at a dry skillet.
Stir-r the beans into the curry and then simmer for two mins. Insert the lettuce in handfuls, allowing each to simmer before adding the following: simmer for 1 minute. Bring the lemon juice, to taste, & the majority of the coriander leaves. Scatter on the remaining coriander and cashews, then use the rice and lemon wedges
Nutrition:
Calories: 747 Carbs: 91g Fat: 37g Protein: 14g

25.   Chicken Liver Along with Tomato Ragu

Preparation Time: 10 minutes
Cooking time: 30 minutes
Servings: 2
Ingredients
2 tbsp. olive oil
1 onion, finely chopped
2 carrots scrubbed and simmer
4 garlic cloves, finely chopped
1/4 x 2 tbsp. pack fresh ginger, stalks finely chopped, leaves ripped
package poultry livers, finely chopped, and almost any sinew removed and lost
2 cups tin grower's harvest chopped berries
1 chicken stock cube, created around 300ml
1/2 tsp caster sugar
1cup penne
1/4 lemon, juiced

Directions:
Heat 1 tablespoon oil in a large skillet, over a low-medium heating system. Fry the onion and carrots to 10 mins, stirring periodically. Stir in the ginger and garlic pops and cook 2 mins more. Transfer into a bowl set aside.

Twist the pan into high heat and then add the oil. Bring the chicken livers and simmer for 5 mins until browned. Pour the onion mix to the pan and then stir in the tomatoes, sugar, and stock. Seasons bring to the boil, and then simmer for 20 mins until reduced and thickened, and the liver is cooked through. Meanwhile, cook pasta to package guidelines.

Taste the ragu and put in a second pinch of sugar more seasoning, if needed. Put in a squeeze of lemon juice to taste and stir in two of the ripped basil leaves. Divide the pasta between four bowls, then spoon across the ragu and top with the rest of the basil.

Nutrition:
Calories: 469g
Protein: 14g
Fat: 0

26.   Minted Lamb with Couscous Salad

Preparation Time: 10 minutes
Cooking time: 10 minutes
Servings: 2
Ingredients
6 tbsp. couscous
1/2 chicken stock block, composed of 4oz.
2 tbsp. pack, refreshing flat-leaf parsley, sliced
3 mint sprigs, leaves picked and sliced
1 tablespoon olive oil
14 tbsp. pack suspended BBQ minted lamb leg beans, de-frosted
14 tbsp. lettuce berries, sliced
1/4 tsp, sliced
1 spring onion, sliced
Pinch of ground cumin
1/2 lemon, zested and juiced
4 tbsp. reduced-fat salad cheese

Directions:
 Place the couscous into a heatproof bowl and then pour on the inventory. Cover and set aside for 10 mins, then fluff with a fork and stir in the herbs.
 Meanwhile, rub a little oil within the lamb steaks and season. Cook to package guidelines then slit.
Mix the tomatoes, cucumber, and spring onion into the couscous with the oil, the cumin, and lemon juice and zest. Crumble on the salad and serve with the bunny.

Nutrition:
Calories: 381g
Protein: 29g
Fat: 10.2g
Carbohydrates: 40.9g

27.   Jack Fruit Tortilla Bowls

Preparation Time: 10 minutes
Cooking time: 15 minutes
Servings: 2
Ingredients
Two sweet corn cobettes
1 red chili, finely chopped
2 teaspoon olive oil
1 lime, juiced
1 tbsp. fresh coriander, chopped, plus extra to garnish
package stained jack fruit in Tex-Mex sauce
14 tbsp. tin kidney beans, drained
8 tbsp. roasted red peppers (in the jar), drained and chopped
Two whitened tortilla packs
1/2 round lettuce, ripped
Directions:
Heat a griddle pan on a high temperature (or light a barbecue). Griddle that the cobettes to get 10 12 mins, turning until cooked and charred throughout. Remove from the pan and stand upright onto a plank. Use a sharp knife to carefully reduce the span of this corn, staying near to the heart, to clear away the kernels. Mix that the kernels with the eucalyptus oil, half of the carrot juice along with half an hour of the coriander.

Heating the jack fruit and sauce in a saucepan with the legumes, peppers, staying lime coriander and juice on medium-low heating for 3-4 mins until heated through.

Griddle the wraps for 10 20 secs each side to char. Tear into pieces and serve together with all the
 jack fruit lettuce and sweet corn salsa.
Nutrition:
Calories 387.
Fat 11g.
Sodium 381mg.
Carbohydrates: 70g.
Fiber 9g.

28.   Carrot, Courgette and Halloumi Hamburgers (Veggie Recipe)

Preparation Time: 10 minutes
Cooking time: 60 minutes
Servings: 2
Ingredients
 1 big carrot, grated
 1 large courgette, grated
8oz. halloumi, grated
 2 spring onions, finely chopped
 3oz. breadcrumbs
0.5 oz. ground cumin
0.5oz. ground coriander
 1/2 teaspoon salt
1 oz. flour
 4 brioche buns, halved
 2 oz. baby spinach leaves
 1 big tomato, sliced
 1 small red onion, chopped
 1/2 pineapple, peeled into ribbons
Tzatziki, to function

Directions:
 Place the courgette into a clean tea towel and squeeze to eradicate any liquid. Hint into a big bowl and then add the carrot, halloumi, onion, breadcrumbs, cumin, coriander, eggs, salt, and flour. Stir well to mix.
 Put only over half the mix in a food processor and pulse until the mixture starts to stay.
 Divide the mix into 4 and then form into patties. Heat a grill or griddle pan into a moderate heat. Cook the hamburgers for 45 mins each side until golden and cooked through. Insert the hamburger buns into the grill till lightly toasted. To assemble the burgers, put lettuce leaves on the base of each bun. Top with the entire hamburger, a piece of tomato, pineapple ribbon along with a spoonful of tzatziki.

Nutrition:
Calories: 937 kcal Fat58.0 g Saturates: 27.0 g Carbohydrate: 62 g Sugars: 14.0 gProtein: 44 gSalt:4.0g

CHAPTER 6:

Juices and Smoothie

29.   Green-Berry Smoothie

Preparation Time: 20 Minutes
Cooking Time: 0 Minutes
Servings 2
Ingredients:
1 ripe banana
½ cup blackcurrants take off stems
10 baby kale leaves take off stems
2 tsp honey
1 cup freshly made green tea dissolve honey first in tea then chill
6 ice cubes
Directions:
Dissolve the honey in the tea before you chill it. Cool first, and then blend all ingredients blender until smooth.
Nutrition:
Calories: 157.9g
Cholesterol: 0
Carbohydrates: 37g

30.   Creamy Strawberry & Cherry Smoothie

Preparation Time: 20 Minutes
Cooking Time: 0 Minutes
Servings 2
Ingredients
100g 3½ oz. strawberries
75g 3oz. frozen pitted cherries
1 tablespoon plain full-fat yogurt
175mls 6fl oz. unsweetened soya milk
132 calories per serving
Directions:
Place all the ingredients into a blender and process until smooth. Serve and enjoy.
Nutrition:
Calories: 138g Carbohydrates: 30g Fat: 0 Protein: 0

31.   Matcha Green Tea Smoothie

Preparation Time: 10 Minutes
Cooking Time: 0 Minutes
Servings 2
Ingredients
2 bananas
2 tsp Matcha green tea powder
1/2 tsp vanilla bean paste or scraped from a vanilla bean pod
1 ½ cups milk
4-5 ice cubes
2 tsp honey
Directions:
Add all ingredients except the Matcha to a blender. Blend until smooth. Sprinkle in the Matcha tea powder, stir well or blend a few seconds more or add cooled green tea).
Nutrition:
Calories: 212g
Carbohydrates: 39g
Protein: 99g

32.   Grape, Celery & Parsley Reviver

Preparation Time: 10 Minutes
Cooking Time: 0 Minutes
Servings 2
Ingredients
75g 3oz red grapes
3 sticks of celery
1 avocado, de-stoned and peeled
1 tablespoon fresh parsley
½ teaspoon matcha powder
334 calories per serving
Directions:
Place all the ingredients into a blender with enough water to cover them and blitz until smooth and creamy. Add crushed ice to make it even more refreshing.
Nutrition:
Calories: 182g
Total Fat: 1.2g
Carbohydrates: 49.9g
Cholesterol: 0

33.   Green Juice Recipe

Preparation Time: 10 Minutes
Cooking Time: 0 Minutes
Servings 2
Ingredients
1 large handful of rockets
Two large handfuls of kale
1 exceedingly small handful of Lovage leaves optional
2 or 3 large stalks of green celery including the leaves
½ medium green apples
Juice of ½ lemon
1 exceedingly small handful of parsley
½ level teaspoon of Matcha
Directions:
 Mix the greens well and juice them to get about 50 ml of juice.
 Juice the apple and the celery, and then peel the lemon and juice it by hand.
Pour a little of the juice in a glass, add matcha powder, and then stir vigorously. Once it has dissolved, pour it back on the juice, and stir it in. Add some water if the blend is a little too strong for you and serve.
Nutrition:
Calories: 83g
Carbohydrates: 20g
Protein: 2g

34.   Strawberry & Citrus Blend

Preparation Time: 20 Minutes
Cooking Time: 0 Minutes
Servings 2
Ingredients
75g 3oz strawberries
1 apple, cored
1 orange, peeled
½ avocado, peeled, and de-stoned
½ teaspoon matcha powder
Juice of 1 lime
272 calories per serving
Directions:
Place all the ingredients into a blender with enough water to cover them and process until smooth.
Nutrition:
Calories: 4.5 g
Total Fat: 2.1 g
Cholesterol: 180 mg
Carbohydrates: 5.3 g
Fiber: 59 g
Sugar: 16.9 g

35.   Grape and Melon Smoothie

Preparation Time: 20 Minutes Cooking Time: 0 Minutes Servings 1
Ingredients
8 tbsp. of cantaloupe melon
8 tbsp. of red seedless grapes
2 tbsp. of young spinach leaves stalks removed
½ cucumber
Directions:
Peel the cucumber, then cut it into half. Remove the seeds and chop them roughly.
Peel the cantaloupe, deseed it, and cut it into chunks.
Place all ingredients in a blender and blend until smooth.
Nutrition:
Calories: 187g Carbohydrates: 52g Fat: 0.1g Protein: 0.2g

36.   Watermelon Juice

Preparation Time: 20 Minutes
Cooking Time: 0 Minutes
Servings 1
Ingredients
1 tbsp. of young kale leaves
1 cup of watermelon chunks
4 mint leaves
½ cucumbers
Directions:
 Remove the stalks from the kale and roughly chop it.
 Peel the cucumber, if preferred, and then halve it and seed it.
Place all ingredients in a blender or juicer and process until you achieve the desired consistency. Serve immediately.
Nutrition:
Calories: 30.g Protein: 0.6 g. Carbohydrates: 7.6 g. Sugar: 6.2 g.
Fiber: 0.4 g. Fat: 0.2 g

37.   Mango & Rocket Arugula Smoothie

Preparation Time: 10 Minutes
Cooking Time: 0 Minutes
Servings 2
Ingredients
25g 1oz fresh rocket arugula
150g 5oz fresh mango, peeled, de-stoned and chopped
1 avocado, de-stoned and peeled
½ teaspoon matcha powder
Juice of 1 lime
369 calories per serving
Directions:
Place all the ingredients into a blender with enough water to cover them and process until smooth. Add a few ice cubes and enjoy.
Nutrition:
Calories: 220g
Sugar: 17g
Fat: 18g
Carbohydrates: 25g
Fiber: 7g
Protein: 3g

38. Green Tea Smoothie

Preparation Time: 20 Minutes
Cooking Time: 0 Minutes
Servings 2
Ingredients
2 teaspoons of honey
250 ml of milk
2 teaspoons of matcha green tea powder 6 ice cubes
½ teaspoon of vanilla bean paste not extractor a scrape of the seeds from the vanilla pod
2 ripe bananas
Directions:
1. Place all the ingredients in a blender and run until you achieve the desired consistency.
2. Serve into two glasses and enjoy.
Nutrition: Saturated Fats: 20g Cholesterol: 300mg Sodium: 2400mg Potassium: 3500mg

39. Berries Banana Smoothie

Preparation Time: 10 Minutes
Cooking Time: 0 Minutes
Servings 2
Ingredients
½ cup of coconut milk
1½ cups of mixed berries strawberries and blueberries) - could be frozen or fresh
¾ cup of water
4 ice cubes
1 tablespoon of molasses
1 banana
Directions:
Place all the ingredients in a blender and blend until smooth.
You can add water to the smoothie until you achieve your desired consistency, and then serve.
 Nutrition:
Calories: 91.7g Cholesterol: 0g Sodium: 2.3mg Carbs:23.3g

CHAPTER 7:

Sirtfood Diet Salads and Dressings

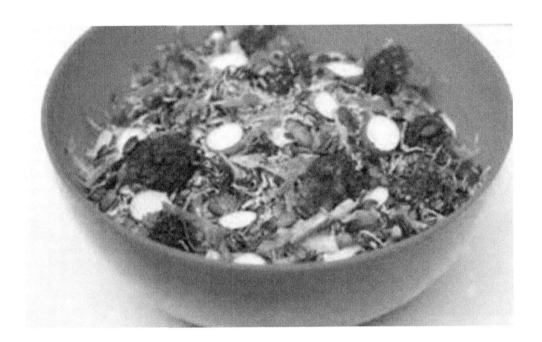

40.   Spring Strawberry Kale Salad

Preparation Time: 5 minutes
Servings: 4
Ingredients
3 cups baby kale, rinsed and dried
10 large strawberries, sliced
½ cup honey
1/3 cup white wine vinegar
1 cup extra virgin olive oil

1 tablespoon poppy seeds
2 tablespoons pine nuts, toasted
Salt and pepper to taste

Directions:

In a large bowl, mix the baby kale with the strawberries.

To make the dressing: In a blender, add the honey, vinegar, and oil and blend until smooth.

Stir in the poppy seeds and season to taste

Pour over the kale and strawberries and toss to coat.

Nutrition:

Calories: 220cal
Carbohydrates: 21g
Fat: 15g
Protein: 5g

41.   Blackberry Arugula Salad

Preparation Time: 5 minutes
Servings: 5
Ingredients
3 cups baby arugula, rinsed and dried
1-pint fresh blackberries
¾ cups of crumbled feta cheese
1-pint cherry tomatoes, halved
1 green onion, sliced
¼ cup walnuts, chopped (optional)
To Serve:
Balsamic reduction, as required
Directions:
 In a large bowl, toss together baby arugula, blackberries, feta cheese, cherry tomatoes, green onion, and walnuts.
Drizzle balsamic reduction over plated salads
Nutrition:
Calories: 270
Fat: 13g
Saturated Fat: 2g
Carbohydrates: 38g

42.   Apple Walnut Spinach Salad

Preparation Time: 5 minutes
Servings: 4
Ingredients
3 cups baby spinach
1 medium apple, chopped
¼ Medjool dates, chopped
¼ cup walnuts, chopped
2 tablespoons extra virgin olive oil
1 tablespoon sugar
1 tablespoon apple cider vinegar
½ teaspoon curry powder
¼ teaspoon turmeric
1/8 teaspoon chili pepper flakes
¼ teaspoon salt
Directions:
In a large bowl, combine the spinach, apple, dates, and walnuts.
To make the dressing: In a jar with a tight-fitting lid, combine the remaining ingredients; shake well.
Drizzle over salad and toss to coat.
Nutrition:
Calories: 166.1
Fat: 11.9g
Cholesterol: 5.0g
Carbohydrates: 12.6g

43.   Enhanced Waldorf salad

Preparation Time: 5 minutes
Servings: 4
Ingredients
4 – 5 stalks celery, sliced
1 medium apple, chopped
¼ cup walnuts, chopped
1 small red onion, diced
1 head of red endive, chopped
2 teaspoons fresh parsley, finely diced
1 tablespoon capers, drained
2 teaspoons Lovage or celery leaves, finely diced
For the dressing:
1 tablespoon extra-virgin olive oil
1 teaspoon balsamic vinegar
1 teaspoon Dijon mustard
Juice of half a lemon
Directions:
To make the dressing: Whisk together the oil, vinegar, mustard, and lemon juice.
Add the remaining salad ingredients to a medium – large-sized salad bowl and toss.
Drizzle the dressing over the salad, mix, and serve cold.
Nutrition:
Calorie: 582Kcal
Fat: 103g
Fat: 22.2g
Protein: 8.2g

44.   Kale Salad with Pepper Jelly Dressing

Preparation Time: 5 minutes
Servings: 4
Ingredients
4 tablespoons mild pepper jelly
3 tablespoons olive oil
¼ teaspoon salt
½ teaspoon Dijon mustard
3 cups baby kale leaves
½ cup goat cheese, crumbled
¼ cup walnuts, chopped
Directions:
To make the dressing: In a small bowl, whisk together the pepper jelly, olive oil, salt, and mustard.
Heat in the microwave for 30 seconds. Let cool.
Place the kale in a large bowl and toss with the dressing. Serve topped with goat cheese and sprinkle with walnuts.
Nutrition:
Calories: 1506.3 Kcal
Cholesterol: 25.3mg
Carbohydrates: 96.3g

45.   Hot Arugula and Artichoke Salad

Preparation Time: 5 minutes
Cooking time: 10 minutes
Servings: 2
Ingredients
1 tablespoon extra-virgin olive oil
2 cups baby arugula, washed and dried
1 red onion, thinly sliced
1 (3/4 cups) jar marinated artichoke hearts, quartered or chopped
1 cup feta cheese, crumbled
Directions:
Preheat oven to 300 degrees F.
Drizzle olive oil on a rimmed baking sheet. Spread arugula in a thick layer covering the baking sheet.
Arrange onions and artichokes over the spinach and drizzle the marinade from the jar over the entire salad.
Sprinkle with the cheese and bake for about 10 minutes, or until the arugula is wilted but NOT crispy.
Serve warm.
Nutrition:
Calories: 281Kcal
Fat: 26.g
Cholesterol: 126mg
Protein: 7g

46.　　Spinach and Chicken Salad

Preparation Time: 5 minutes
Servings: 4
Ingredients
2 cups fresh spinach, rinsed and dried
4 cooked skinless, boneless chicken breast halves, sliced
1 zucchini, halved lengthwise and sliced
1 red bell pepper, chopped
½ cup black olives
¼ cup capers, drained
½ cups fontina cheese, frozen and shredded
Directions:
Place equal portions of spinach onto four salad plates.
Arrange chicken, zucchini, bell pepper, and black olives and capers over spinach and top with
Cheese.
Nutrition:
Calories: 120
Fat: 4.9g
Cholesterol: 15mg
Carbohydrates: 13g

47.   Warm Citrus Chicken Salad

Preparation Time: 10 minutes
Servings: 4
Ingredients
3 cups torn fresh kale
2 mandarin oranges, peeled and pulled into individual segments
½ cup mushrooms, sliced
1 small red onion, sliced
½ pound skinless, boneless chicken breast halves - cut into strips
¼ cup walnuts, chopped
2 tablespoons extra virgin olive oil
2 teaspoons cornstarch
½ teaspoon ground ginger
¼ cup pure orange juice, fresh squeezed is best
¼ cup red wine vinegar or apple cider vinegar
Directions:
The place was torn kale, orange segments, mushrooms, and onion into a large bowl and toss to combine.
 In a skillet, sauté chicken and walnuts in oil stirring frequently until chicken is no longer pink, a minimum of 10 minutes.
In a small bowl, whisk the cornstarch, ginger, orange juice, and vinegar until smooth.
Stir into the chicken mixture. Bring to a boil and simmer, continually stirring for 2 minutes or until thickened and bubbly.
Serve salads and pour chicken mixture over the top.
Nutrition:
Calories: 237
Fat: 11.3g
Carbohydrates: 9.8g
Cholesterol: 101.9mg

48.　　Summer Buckwheat Salad

Preparation Time: 15 minutes
Cooking time: 30 minutes
Servings: 4
Ingredients
½ cup buckwheat groats
¾ cup corn kernels
2 medium-sized carrots, diced
1 spring onion, diced
¼ cucumber, chopped
1 red onion, diced
10 radishes, chopped
3 cups cooked black beans
Directions:
Using a fine-mesh sieve, rinse the buckwheat under running water
Bring to a boil in 1 cup of water, and then reduce to a simmer, covered, for 10 minutes
Drain well and chill in the fridge for at least 30 minutes
Combine cooled buckwheat and remaining ingredients in a large salad bowl
Nutrition:
Calories: 128
Fat: 22g
Protein: 4g

49.   Greek-Style Shrimp Salad on a Bed of Baby Kale

Preparation Time: 15 minutes
Servings: 4
Ingredients
1-pound raw shrimp (26 to 30), peeled
¼ cup extra virgin olive oil plus more, as needed for grilling
Salt and pepper to taste
Sugar to taste
2 medium tomatoes, diced
½ cup feta cheese, crumbled
½ cup black olives, sliced
1 teaspoon dried oregano
4 teaspoons red wine vinegar
3 cups of baby kale
Directions:
Preheat a gas grill or barbeque on high.
Thread shrimp onto metal skewers (or bamboo ones that have been soaked in water for 15 minutes).
Brush both sides with oil and season with salt, pepper, and sugar, to taste.
Grill shrimp until fully cooked and spotty brown, about 2 minutes per side.
Meanwhile, in a medium-sized bowl, combine the tomatoes, cheese, olives, oregano, 2 tablespoons. Of the olive oil and 2 teaspoons of the vinegar.
When the shrimp is cooked, unthread it carefully and add to bowl. Lightly toss all the ingredients to coat. Set aside.
When ready to serve, drizzle remaining oil over kale in a large bowl, tossing to coat. Add remaining vinegar and toss again.
Divide kale among 4 large plates. Top each with a portion of the shrimp mixture.
Nutrition:
Calories: 460
Carbohydrates: 13g
Fat: 33g
Protein: 30g

50. Walnut Herb Pesto

Preparation Time: 5 minutes
Servings: 4-6
Ingredients
1 cup walnuts
¾ cup parsley, chopped
¾ cup Lovage, chopped
¾ cup basil, chopped
½ cup Parmesan, grated
3 cloves of garlic, chopped
½ teaspoon salt
½ cup extra virgin olive oil
Directions:
Combine all ingredients except olive oil in a food processor and pulse for a few seconds to combine. You may need to scrape down the sides a few times to get the mixture well pureed.
Drizzle in the olive oil while the machine is running to incorporate the oil – don't over the process once the oil is added, 30 seconds is plenty
Serve with crisped baguette slices or pasta
Nutrition:
Calories: 31
Fat: 3.1g
Carbohydrates: 0.8g

51. Creamy Lovage Dressing

Preparation Time: 5 minutes
Servings: 2-3
Ingredients
1 lemon, juiced
1 teaspoon garlic powder
1 teaspoon dried onion powder
1 teaspoon Dijon mustard
1 teaspoon Lovage
¼ cup walnuts, soaked
1 teaspoon date or maple syrup
Salt and pepper to taste
Directions:
Blend the soaked nuts with the date syrup to make walnut butter.
Place all ingredients in a small mixing bowl.
Whisk well to combine.
Nutrition:
 Calories: 90Kcal
Carbohydrates: 6g
Fat: 8g
Protein:0

CHAPTER 8:

Sirtfood Diet Snacks and Desserts

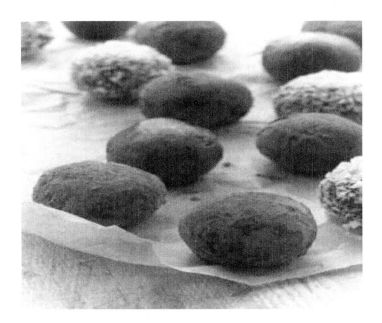

52.　　Maple Walnut Cupcakes with Matcha Green Tea Icing

Preparation Time: 20 minutes
Cooking time: 25 minutes
Servings: 4
Ingredients
For the Cupcakes:
2 cups of All-Purpose flour
½ cup buckwheat flour
2 ½ teaspoons baking powder

½ teaspoon salt
1 cup of cocoa butter
1 cup white sugar
1 tablespoon pure maple syrup
3 eggs
1 teaspoon maple extract
2/3 cup milk
· ¼ cup walnuts, chopped

For the Icing:
 3 tablespoons coconut oil, thick at room temperature
 3 tablespoons icing sugar
 1 tablespoon Matcha green tea powder
 ½ teaspoon vanilla bean paste
 3 tablespoons cream cheese, softened

Directions:
Preheat oven to 350 degrees F.
Place paper baking cups into muffin tins for 24 regular-sized muffins.
In a medium bowl, mix flours, baking powder, and salt.
In a separate large bowl, cream the sugar, butter, syrup, and eggs with a hand or stand mixer.
Pause to stir in maple extract.
 On low speed, alternate blending in dry mixture and milk.
Fold in nuts.
Pour batter into muffin cup until 2/3 full.
Bake for 20-25 minutes or until an inserted toothpick comes out clean.
Cool completely before icing.
To Make the Icing: Add the coconut oil and icing sugar to a bowl and use a hand-mixer to cream until it's pale and smooth.
Fold in the matcha powder and vanilla.
Finally, add the cream cheese and beat until smooth.
Pipe or spread over the cupcakes once they're cool.

Nutrition:
Calories: 160
Fat: 21g
Carbohydrates: 6g
Protein: 2g

53.   Garlic Lovers Hummus

Preparation Time: 5 minutes
Cooking time: 10 minutes
Servings: 4
Ingredients:
3 tbsps. Freshly squeezed lemon juice
All-purpose salt-free seasoning
3 tbsps. Sesame tahini
4 garlic cloves
15 oz. no-salt-added garbanzo beans
2 tbsps. Olive oil
Directions:
Drain garbanzo beans and rinse thoroughly.
Place all the ingredients in a food processor and pulse until smooth.
Serve immediately or cover and refrigerate until serving.
Nutrition:
Calories: 40g
Carbohydrates: 5g
Fat: 1g
Protein: 2g

54.   Endive Leaves with Citrus Cream

Preparation Time: 15 minutes
Cooking time: 30 minutes
Servings: 4
Ingredients
4-6 heads Red endive
¾ cup cream cheese
1 tablespoon shallot, finely chopped
¼ cup sour cream
¼ cup Vegannaise or mayonnaise
Zest from one small lemon
1 tablespoon lemon juice
2 tablespoons fresh tarragon, chopped
2 tablespoons fresh dill, chopped, plus extra for garnish if desired
2 tablespoons parsley, chopped
1 tablespoon green onions, finely chopped
Anchovy paste (optional), to taste
Salt and pepper, to taste
Directions:
In a medium bowl, whisk all ingredients together, except the endive leaves, until smooth. Refrigerate until needed.
When well chilled, place filling into a piping bag with a French tip.
Trim the stem end of the endive leaves and carefully peel the leaves off the base of the head, so you have individual leaves.
Place the leaves in a single layer on a platter and fill with the cream from the piping bag. Alternatively, spoon the filling into a small bowl or ramekin and serve the endive leaves and crackers around it for guests to help themselves.
Nutrition:
Calories: 478
Carbohydrates: 8g
Protein: 29g

55.   Greek Stuffed Mushrooms

Preparation Time: 10 minutes
Cooking time: 20 minutes
Servings: 4
Ingredients
20 large mushrooms, washed
1 tablespoon extra-virgin olive oil
1 cup broccoli, chopped
1 medium red onion, diced
1 teaspoon garlic, minced
¼ cup capers
½ teaspoon dried oregano
½ teaspoon dried parsley
3 tablespoons feta cheese
1 tablespoon breadcrumbs
Salt and pepper to taste

Directions:
Preheat oven to 425 degrees F.
Remove the stems from the mushrooms carefully and dice them.
Place mushroom tops in a single layer on a baking sheet, with the hole facing up, and bake for 5 minutes.
Head olive oil in a pan with the diced mushrooms stems, broccoli, onion, garlic, capers, oregano, parsley and salt, and pepper. Cook for 5 – 10 minutes.
Add feta and breadcrumbs.
Stuff mushrooms with mixture and bake for 8 – 10 minutes.

Nutrition:
Calories: 287
 Fat: 11.2g,
Carbohydrates: 9.6g,
Protein: 15.3g

56.   Roast Tomato and Parmesan Bruschetta with Capers

Preparation Time: 5 minutes
Cooking time: 10 minutes
Servings: 4
Ingredients
 4 to 6 thick slices of whole-grain baguette, sliced on a diagonal
 1 cup cherry tomatoes
 2 tablespoons capers, drained
 3 to 4 tablespoons extra virgin olive oil + 1 tablespoon extra
 ½ teaspoon of sea salt
 2/3 cup aged Parmesan, shaved
Directions:
Preheat oven to 400 degrees F.

Mix the cherry tomatoes, capers, and 3 to 4 tablespoons of olive oil and pour into an ovenproof dish—roast for 10 to 15 minutes.

While the tomatoes are roasting, toast the bread on both sides and drizzle the remaining 1 tablespoon of oil over the dough.

Spoon the roast tomatoes and capers over the toasted bread, salt to taste, and top with the shaved Parmesan to serve.

Nutrition:
Calories: 39
Carbohydrates: 6.1g
Protein: 32g
Cholesterol: 0.6

57. Chocolate Maple Walnuts

Preparation Time: 15 minutes
Cooking time: 30 minutes
Servings: 4
Ingredients
½ cup pure maple syrup, divided
2 cups raw, whole walnuts
5 squares of dark chocolate, at least 85%
1 ½ tablespoons coconut oil, melted
1 tablespoonful of water
Sifted icing sugar
1 teaspoonful of vanilla extract
Directions:
Line a large baking sheet with parchment paper.
In a medium to a large skillet, combine the walnuts and ¼ cup of maple syrup and cook over medium heat, stirring continuously, until walnuts are completely covered with syrup and golden in color, about 3 – 5 minutes.
Pour the walnuts onto the parchment paper and separate it into individual pieces with a fork. Allow cooling completely; at least 15 minutes.
In the meantime, melt the chocolate in a double boiler with the coconut oil. Add the remaining maple syrup and stir until thoroughly combined.
When walnuts are cooled, transfer them to a glass bowl and pour the melted chocolate syrup over the top. Use a silicone spatula to mix until walnuts are completely covered gently.
Transfer back to the parchment paper-lined baking sheet and, once again, separate each of the nuts with a fork.
Place the nuts in the fridge for 10 minutes or the freezer for 3 – 5 minutes, until chocolate has completely set.
Store in an airtight bag in your fridge.
Nutrition Facts per Serving
Calories: 249
Sugar: 20g
Fat: 16g
Cholesterol: 28g

58.   Matcha and Chocolate Dipped Strawberries

Preparation Time: 5 minutes
Cooking time: 10 minutes
 Servings: 4
Ingredients
 4 tablespoons cocoa butter
 4 squares of dark chocolate, at least 85%
 ¼ cup of coconut oil
 1 teaspoon Matcha green tea powder
 20 – 25 large whole strawberries, stems on
Directions:
Melt cocoa butter, dark chocolate, coconut oil, and Matcha in a double boiler until nearly smooth.
Remove from heat and continue stirring until chocolate is completely melted.
Pour into a large glass bowl and continuously stir until the chocolate thickens and starts to lose its sheen, about 2 - 5 minutes.
Working one at a time, hold the strawberries by stems and dip into chocolate matcha mixture to coat. Let excess drip back into the bowl.
Place on a parchment-lined baking sheet and chill dipped berries in the fridge until the shell is set, 20–25 minutes.
You may need to reheat matcha mixture if it starts to set before you have dipped all the berries.
Nutrition Facts per Serving
Calories: 88.1
Fat: 5.3g
Cholesterol: 0
Sugar: 9.8g

59.   Vegan Rice Pudding

Preparation Time: 10 minutes
Cooking time: 20 minutes |
Servings: 3
Ingredients:
½ tsp. ground cinnamon
1 c. rinsed basmati
1/8 tsp. ground cardamom
¼ c. sugar
1/8 tsp. pure almond extract
1-quart vanilla nondairy milk
1 tsp. pure vanilla extract
Directions:
Measure all the ingredients into a saucepan and stir well to combine. Bring to a boil over medium-high heat.
Once boiling, reduce heat to low and simmer, stirring very frequently, about 15–20 minutes.
Remove from heat and cool. Serve sprinkled with additional ground cinnamon if desired.
Nutrition Facts per Serving
Calories: 148
Fat: 2 g
Carbohydrates: 26 g
Protein: 4 g
Sugars: 35 g,

60.   Cinnamon-Scented Quinoa

Preparation Time: 5 minutes
Cooking time: 10 minutes
Servings: 4
 Ingredients:

Chopped walnuts
1 ½ c. water
Maple syrup
2 cinnamon sticks
1 c. quinoa

Directions:

Add the quinoa to a bowl and wash it in several changes of water until the water is clear. When washing quinoa, rub grains and allow them to settle before you pour off the water.

Use a large fine-mesh sieve to drain the quinoa. Prepare your pressure cooker with a trivet and steaming basket. Place the quinoa, and the cinnamon sticks in the basket and pour the water.

Close and lock the lid. Cook at high pressure for 6 minutes. When the cooking time is up, release the pressure using the quick release Directions:

Fluff the quinoa with a fork and remove the cinnamon sticks. Divide the cooked quinoa among serving bowls and top with maple syrup and chopped walnuts.

Nutrition:

Calories: 160
 Fat: 3 g
Carbohydrates: 28 g
Protein: 6 g
Sugars: 19 g
Sodium:40mg

CHAPTER 9:

Sirtfood Diet Main Meals

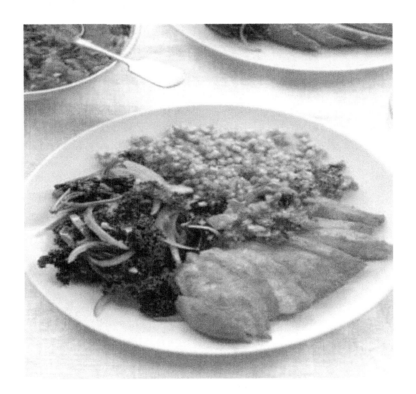

61.   Coq Au Vin

Preparation Time: 10 minutes
Cooking time: 1hr and 15 minutes
Servings: 8
Ingredients
450g (1lb) button mushrooms
100g (3½oz) streaky bacon, chopped

16 chicken thighs, skin removed
3 cloves of garlic, crushed
3 tablespoons fresh parsley, chopped
3 carrots, chopped
2 red onions, chopped
2 tablespoons plain flour
2 tablespoons olive oil
750mls (1¼ pints) red wine
1 bouquet garnish

Directions:

Place the flour on a large plate and coat the chicken in it. Heat the olive oil in a large saucepan, add the chicken and brown it, before setting aside. Fry the bacon in the pan, then add the onion and cook for 5 minutes. Pour in the red wine and add the chicken, carrots, bouquet garni, and garlic. Transfer it to a large ovenproof dish. Cook in the oven at 180C/360F for 1 hour. Remove the bouquet garni and skim off any excess fat, if necessary. Add in the mushrooms and cook for 15 minutes. Stir in the parsley just before serving.

Nutrition:

Calories: 267
Fat: 8.7g
Cholesterol: 77.6
Protein: 31.2

62.   Turkey Satay Skewers

Preparation Time: 10 minutes
Cooking time: 10 minutes
Servings: 2
Ingredients
250g (9oz) turkey breast, cubed
25g (1oz) smooth peanut butter
1 clove of garlic, crushed
½ small bird's eye chili (or more if you like it hotter), finely chopped
½ teaspoon ground turmeric
200mls (7fl oz.) coconut milk
2 teaspoons soy sauce
Directions:
Combine the coconut milk, peanut butter, turmeric, soy sauce, garlic, and chili. Add the turkey pieces to the bowl and stir them until they are completely coated. Push the turkey onto metal skewers. Place the satay skewers on a barbeque or under a hot grill (broiler) and cook for 4-5 minutes on each side, until they are completely cooked.
Nutrition:
Calories: 414
Carbohydrates: 6g
Fat: 12g
Protein: 66g

63.   Salmon & Capers

Preparation Time: 10 minutes
Cooking time: 10 minutes
Servings: 4
Ingredients
75g (3oz) Greek yogurt
4 salmon fillets, skin removed
4 teaspoons Dijon Mustard
1 tablespoon capers, chopped
2 teaspoons fresh parsley
Zest of 1 lemon
Directions:
In a bowl, mix the yogurt, mustard, lemon zest, parsley, and capers. Thoroughly coat the salmon in the mixture. Place the salmon under a hot grill (broiler) and cook for 3-4 minutes on each side or until the fish is cooked. Serve with mashed potatoes and vegetables or a large green leafy salad.
Nutrition:
Calories: 430
Carbohydrates: 3g
Fat: 24g
Protein: 45g

64.   Moroccan Chicken Casserole

Preparation Time: 10 minutes
Cooking time: 10 minutes
Servings: 4
Ingredients
250g (9oz) tinned chickpeas (garbanzo beans) drained
4 chicken breasts, cubed
4 Medjool dates halved
6 dried apricots, halved
1 red onion, sliced
1 carrot, chopped
1 teaspoon ground cumin
1 teaspoon ground cinnamon
1 teaspoon ground turmeric
1 bird's-eye chili, chopped
600mls (1 pint) chicken stock (broth)
25g (1oz) corn flour
60mls (2fl oz.) water
2 tablespoons fresh coriander
Directions:
Place the chicken, chickpeas (garbanzo beans), onion, carrot, chili, cumin, turmeric, cinnamon, and stock (broth) into a large saucepan. Bring it to the boil, reduce the heat and simmer for 25 minutes. Add in the dates and apricots and simmer for 10 minutes. In a cup, mix the corn flour with the water until it becomes a smooth paste. Pour the mixture into the saucepan and stir until it thickens. Add in the coriander (cilantro) and mix well. Serve with buckwheat or couscous.
Nutrition:
Calories: 283
Carbohydrates: 26g
Fat: 6g
Protein: 30g

65.   Chili Con Carne

Preparation Time: 10 minutes

Cooking time: 40 minutes

Servings: 4

Ingredients
450g (1lb) lean minced beef
400g (14oz) chopped tomatoes
200g (7oz) red kidney beans
2 tablespoons tomato purée
2 cloves of garlic, crushed
2 red onions, chopped
2 birds-eye chilies, finely chopped
1 red pepper (bell pepper), chopped
1 stick of celery, finely chopped
1 tablespoon cumin
1 tablespoon turmeric
1 tablespoon cocoa powder
400mls (14 fl oz.) beef stock (broth)
175mls (6fl oz.) red wine
1 tablespoon olive oil

Directions:
Heat the oil in a large saucepan, add the onion and cook for 5 minutes. Add in the garlic, celery, chili, turmeric, and cumin and cook for 2 minutes before adding then meat then cook for another 5 minutes. Pour in the stock (broth), red wine, tomatoes, tomato purée, red pepper (bell pepper), kidney beans, and cocoa powder. Simmer on a low heat for 45 minutes, keep it covered, and stirring occasionally. Serve with brown rice or buckwheat.

Nutrition:
Calories: 551
Carbohydrates: 32g
Fat: 108g
Protein: 42g

66.   Prawn & Coconut Curry

Preparation Time: 10 minutes
Cooking time: 5 minutes
Servings: 4
Ingredients
400g (14oz) tinned chopped tomatoes
400g (14oz) large prawns (shrimps), shelled and raw
25g (1oz) fresh coriander (cilantro) chopped
3 red onions, finely chopped
3 cloves of garlic, crushed
2 bird's eye chilies
½ teaspoon ground coriander (cilantro)
½ teaspoon turmeric
400mls (14fl oz.) coconut milk
1 tablespoon olive oil
Juice of 1 lime
Directions:
Place the onions, garlic, tomatoes, chilies, lime juice, turmeric, ground coriander (cilantro), chilies and half of the fresh coriander (cilantro) into a blender and blitz until you have a smooth curry paste. Heat the olive oil in a frying pan, add the paste and cook for 2 minutes. Stir in the coconut milk and warm it thoroughly. Add the prawns (shrimps) to the paste and cook them until they have turned pink and are completely cooked. Stir in the fresh coriander (cilantro). Serve with rice.
Nutrition:
Calories: 239.6
Carbohydrates: 9.2g
Fat: 10.7g
Protein: 25.3g

67.   Chicken & Bean Casserole

Preparation Time: 10 minutes
Cooking time: 45 minutes
Servings: 4
Ingredients
400g (14oz) chopped tomatoes
400g (14oz) tinned cannellini beans or haricot beans
8 chicken thighs, skin removed
2 carrots, peeled and finely chopped
2 red onions, chopped
4 sticks of celery
4 large mushrooms
2 red peppers (bell peppers), de-seeded and chopped
1 clove of garlic
2 tablespoons soy sauce
1 tablespoon olive oil
1.75 liters (3 pints) chicken stock (broth)
Directions:
Heat the olive oil in a saucepan, add the garlic and onions and cook for 5 minutes. Add in the chicken and cook for 5 minutes, then add the carrots, cannellini beans, celery, red peppers (bell peppers), and mushrooms. Pour in the stock (broth) soy sauce and tomatoes. Bring it to the boil, reduce the heat and simmer for 45 minutes. Serve with rice or new potatoes
Nutrition:
Calories: 209.1
Carbohydrates: 6.2 g
Fat: 6.6 g
Protein: 31.10 g

68.   Mussels in Red Wine Sauce

Preparation Time: 10 minutes
Cooking time: 5 minutes
Servings: 2
Ingredients
800g (2lb) mussels
2 x 400g (14oz) tins of chopped tomatoes
25g (1oz) butter
1 tablespoon fresh chives, chopped
1 tablespoon fresh parsley, chopped
1 bird's-eye chili, finely chopped
4 cloves of garlic, crushed
400mls (14fl oz.) red wine
Juice of 1 lemon
Directions:
Wash the mussels, remove their beards, and set them aside. Heat the butter in a large saucepan and add in the red wine. Reduce the heat and add the parsley, chives, chili, and garlic whilst stirring. Add in the tomatoes, lemon juice, and mussels. Cover the saucepan and cook for 2-3. Remove the saucepan from the heat and take out any mussels which haven't opened and discard them. Serve and eat immediately.
Nutrition:
Calories: 388.9
Carbohydrates: 18.0g
Fat: 15. g
Protein: 37.2 g

69.   Roast Balsamic Vegetables

Preparation Time: 10 minutes
Cooking time: 45 minutes
Servings: 4
Ingredients
4 tomatoes, chopped
2 red onions, chopped
3 sweet potatoes, peeled and chopped
100g (3½ oz.) red chicory (or if unavailable, use yellow)
100g (3½ oz.) kale, finely chopped
300g (11oz) potatoes, peeled and chopped
5 stalks of celery, chopped
1 bird's-eye chili, de-seeded and finely chopped
2 tablespoons fresh parsley, chopped
2 tablespoons fresh coriander (cilantro) chopped
3 tablespoons olive oil
2 tablespoons balsamic vinegar
1 teaspoon mustard
Sea salt
Freshly ground black pepper
Directions:
Place the olive oil, balsamic, mustard, parsley, and coriander (cilantro) into a bowl and mix well. Toss all the remaining ingredients into the dressing and season with salt and pepper. Transfer the vegetables to an ovenproof dish and cook in the oven at 200C/400F for 45 minutes.
Nutrition:
Calories: 63.8
Carbohydrates: 9.5g
Fat: 2.4 g
Protein: 1.8 g

70. Tomato & Goat's Cheese Pizza

Preparation Time: 10 minutes
Cooking time: 20 minutes
Servings: 2
Ingredients
225g (8oz) buckwheat flour
2 teaspoons dried yeast
Pinch of salt
150mls (5fl oz.) slightly water
1 teaspoon olive oil
For the Topping:
75g (3oz) feta cheese, crumbled
75g (3oz) passata (or tomato paste)
1 tomato, sliced
1 red onion, finely chopped
25g (1oz) rocket (arugula) leaves, chopped

Directions:
In a bowl, combine all the ingredients for the pizza dough then allow it to stand for at least an hour until it has doubled in size. Roll the dough out to a size to suit you. Spoon the passata onto the base and add the rest of the toppings. Bake in the oven at 200C/400F for 15-20 minutes or until browned at the edges and crispy and serve.

Nutrition:
Calories: 480
Carbohydrates: 53gg
Fat: 2.4 g
Protein: 14 g
Cholesterol: 25mg

71. Tofu Thai Curry

Preparation Time: 10 minutes
Cooking time: 5 minutes
Servings: 4
 Ingredients

400g (14oz) tofu, diced
200g (7oz) sugar snaps peas
5cm (2 inches) chunk fresh ginger root, peeled and finely chopped
2 red onions, chopped
2 cloves of garlic, crushed
2 bird's eye chilies
2 tablespoons tomato puree
1 stalk of lemongrass, inner stalks only
1 tablespoon fresh coriander (cilantro), chopped
1 teaspoon cumin
300mls (½ pint) coconut milk
200mls (7fl oz.) vegetable stock (broth)
1 tablespoon virgin olive oil
Juice of 1 lime
 Directions:
Heat the oil in a frying pan, add the onion and cook for 4 minutes. Add in the chilies, cumin, ginger, and garlic and cook for 2 minutes. Add the tomato puree, lemongrass, sugar-snap peas, lime juice, and tofu and cook for 2 minutes. Pour in the stock (broth), coconut milk and coriander (cilantro) and simmer for 5 minutes. Serve with brown rice or buckwheat, and a handful of rockets (arugula) leaves on the side.
Nutrition:
Calories: 210
Carbohydrates: 53gg
Fat: 11 g
Protein: 12.9 g
Cholesterol: 0

72.   Tender Spiced Lamb

Preparation Time: 10 minutes
Cooking time: 4 Hours
Servings: 8
Ingredients
1.35kg (3lb) lamb shoulder
3 red onions, sliced
3 cloves of garlic, crushed
1 bird's eye chili, finely chopped
1 teaspoon turmeric
1 teaspoon ground cumin
½ teaspoon ground coriander (cilantro)
¼ teaspoon ground cinnamon
2 tablespoons olive oil
Directions:
In a bowl, combine the chili, garlic, and spices with a tablespoon of olive oil.
Coat the lamb with the spice mixture and marinate it for an hour, or
overnight if you can. Heat the remaining oil in a pan, add the lamb and
brown it for 3-4 minutes on all sides to seal it. Place the lamb in an ovenproof
dish. Add in the red onions and cover the bowl with foil. Transfer to the oven
and roast at 170C/325F for 4 hours. The lamb should be extremely tender
and falling off the bone. Serve with rice or couscous, salad, or vegetables.
Nutrition:
Calories: 473.2
Carbohydrates: 11.3g
Fat: 16.9g
Protein: 49.2 g
Cholesterol: 145.2mg

73.   Chili Cod Fillets

Preparation Time: 10 minutes
Cooking time: 10 minutes
Servings: 4
Ingredients
4 cod fillets (approx. 150g each)
2 tablespoons fresh parsley, chopped
2 bird's-eye chilies (or more if you like it hot)
2 cloves of garlic, chopped
4 tablespoons olive oil
Directions:
Heat a tablespoon of olive oil in a frying pan, add the fish and cook for 7-8 minutes or until thoroughly cooked, turning once halfway through. Remove and keep warm. Pour the remaining olive oil into the pan and add the chili, chopped garlic, and parsley. Warm it thoroughly. Serve the fish onto plates and pour the warm chili oil over it.
Nutrition:
Calories: 100
Carbohydrates: 0
Fat: 0.5
Protein: 22g
Cholesterol:0

CHAPTER 10:

Sirtfood Diet Appetizer

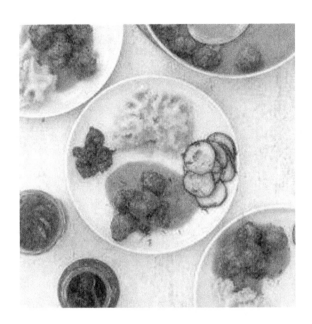

74.   Broccoli Cheddar Bites

Preparation Time: 10 minutes
Cooking time: 30 minutes
Servings: 24 bites
Ingredients:
  1 large bunch of broccoli florets
  ½ cup, packed, torn fresh bread
  2 eggs, lightly beaten
  ¼ cup mayonnaise
  ¼ cup grated onion

1 ½ teaspoons lemon zest
1 cup, packed, grated sharp cheddar cheese
¼ teaspoons freshly ground black pepper
½ teaspoon kosher salt

Directions:

Place 1 inch of water in a pot with a steamer basket. Bring to a boil. Add the broccoli florets. Steam the broccoli florets for 5 minutes, until just tender. Rinse with cold water to stop the cooking. Finely chop the steamed broccoli florets. You should have 2 to 2 ½ cups.

Place the beaten eggs and the torn bread in a large bowl. Mix until the bread is completely moistened. Add the grated onion, mayonnaise, cheese, lemon zest, salt, and pepper. Stir in the minced broccoli.

Preheat the oven to 350° F. Coat the wells of 2 mini muffin pans with olive oil. Distribute the broccoli mixture in the muffin wells.

Bake at 350° F for 25 minutes until cooked through and lightly browned on top. If you don't have mini muffin pans, you can cook the bites freeform. Just grease a baking sheet and spoon large dollops of the mixture onto the pan. Baking time is the same.

Nutrition:

Calories 62 at 4.8g,Carbohydrates 3g,Protein 1.7g

75.   No-Bake Zucchini Roll-Ups

Preparation Time: 10 minutes
Cooking time: 10 minutes
Servings: 20 rolls-up
Ingredients:
 1 large zucchini
 1 jar pepperoncini
 1 medium carrot
 Handful mixed greens
 1 tub guacamole
 1 single celery stalk
 Fresh dill
Directions:
 Using a peeler slice the zucchini the long way, on all sides to avoid the center. Basically, make 3-4 slices on one side and move on to the opposite side, then the other two sides until you have about 20 slices. Don't discard the middle; just add to your next skillet meal. Set aside.
 Using a mandolin slicer, cut the carrots and celery into thin strips. Set aside.
 Finally, cut the top part off each pepperoncino, cut one side to open and clean seeds out.
Arranging the Roll-Ups:
 On a flat surface, place one zucchini stip. spread a dab of guacamole on one end. Place pepperoncini on top of the guacamole, open side up. Fill pocket whole of the pepperoncini with guacamole. Add in 1-2 mixed green leaves, 3 strips of carrots, 1-2 strips of celery, fresh dill, and roll it tight until you reach the end of the zucchini. If you need help keeping the zucchini roll-ups tight in place, add another dab of guacamole on the end part of the zucchini to stick together.
Do this step until you've used all the ingredients.
 Serve cold and refrigerate leftover for up to 24 hours. The guacamole will darken after this time.
Nutrition:
Calories 214
Fat 4.7g
Carbohydrates 4g
Protein 5g

76.   Avocado Deviled Eggs

Preparation Time: 10 minutes
Cooking time: 10 minutes
Servings: 3
Ingredients:
 3 eggs
 1 avocado
1 tablespoon chopped chives
1 tablespoon freshly squeezed lime juice
Directions:
 Peel your hard-boiled eggs and cut them in half, lengthways.
 Remove the cooked yolk and add to a mixing bowl along with the avocado and lime juice.
 Mash, with a fork, until you achieve the desired texture. Stir in the chopped chives.
 Either spoon the mixture back into the eggs or pipe it into the eggs using a piping bag or zip lock again.
 Serve straight away.
Nutrition:
Calories 156,
 Fat 5.3g
Carbohydrates 3.8g
Protein 3.4g

77.   Spicy Deviled Eggs

Preparation Time: 10 minutes
Cooking time: 2 Hours
Servings: 24
Ingredients:
 12 large eggs
 1 tablespoon sriracha sauce
 1/3 cup mayonnaise
 1 tablespoon Dijon mustard
 Fine chili flakes
 Fresh chives, minced
 Salt and freshly ground black pepper to taste

Directions:
 Fill a saucepan with enough water to cover eggs by an inch and bring to a full boil. Carefully lower eggs into boiling water. Let eggs boil uncovered for about 30 seconds. Reduce heat to low and cover. Simmer for 11 minutes. Transfer boiled eggs to a bowl of ice water. When cool enough to handle, gently break shell apart and peel. If possible, refrigerate eggs overnight, making them easier to cut.

 Once eggs are cool, cut in half lengthwise with a very sharp knife. Carefully spoon yolks out into a small bowl and arrange whites on serving platter.

 In a medium bowl, mash yolks into a paste with the back of a fork. Add mayonnaise, sriracha sauce, and mustard, whisk until smooth. Season to taste with salt, freshly ground black pepper and more sriracha if you like.

 Spoon or pipe filling into egg white halves.

 Cover and refrigerate eggs for 2 hours or more (up to 1 day). Once chilled sprinkle generously with fine chili flakes and minced chives. Serve and enjoy!

Nutrition:
Calories 53,
Fat 4g
Carbohydrates: 0.6g
Protein 2 g

78.   Spicy Roasted Nut

Preparation Time: 10 minutes
Cooking time: 10 minutes
Servings: 6
Ingredients:
8 oz. pecans or almonds or walnuts
1 tablespoon olive oil or coconut oil
1 teaspoon paprika powder or chili powder
1 teaspoon ground cumin
1 teaspoon salt
Directions:
Mix all ingredients in a medium frying pan and cook on medium heat until the almonds are warmed through.
Let cool and serve as a snack with a drink. Store in a container with a lid at room temperature.
Nutritional info per serving: Calories 201, Fat 7g, Carbohydrates 5g, Protein 4g
Nutrition:
Calories 201,
 Fat 7g
Carbohydrates 5g
Protein 4g

79.   Crab Salad Stuffed Avocado

Preparation Time: 10 minutes
Cooking time: 10 minutes
Servings: 2
Ingredients:
4 oz. lump crab meat
2 tablespoons light mayonnaise
1 teaspoon chopped fresh chives
¼ cup peeled and diced cucumber
2 teaspoons sriracha, plus more for drizzling
1 small avocado (about 4 oz. avocado when pitted and peeled)
½ teaspoon furikake
2 teaspoons gluten-free soy sauce
Directions:
In a medium bowl, combine mayonnaise, sriracha, and chives.
Add crab meat, cucumber, and chive and gently toss.
Cut the avocado open, remove pit and peel the skin or spoon the avocado out.
Fill the avocado halves equally with crab salad.
Top with furikake and drizzle with soy sauce.
Nutrition:
Calories 194
 Fat 13g
Carbohydrates 7g
 Protein 12g

80.   Cheddar Olives

Preparation Time: 10 minutes
Cooking time: 20 minutes
Servings: 6-8
Ingredients:
1 8-10 jar pitted olives, either pimento-stuffed or plain
1 cup all-purpose flour
1 ½ cups shredded sharp cheddar cheese
¼ teaspoon freshly grated black pepper
4 tablespoons unsalted butter, softened
Directions:
Preheat oven to 400° F. Drain the olives well and dry them completely with clean dish towels. Set aside.
Combine the cheese, flour, butter, and spices in a medium bowl and knead it within the bowl until a dough form. If the dough is still crumbly and won't hold together, add water 1 teaspoon at a time until it does.
Pinch of a small amount of dough and press it as thin as you can between your fingers to flatten. Wrap and smoosh the dough around a dry olive. Pinch off any excess, and then roll the olive in your hands until smooth. Continue until all the olives are covered.
Bake for 15-20 minutes, or until golden brown all over. Serve immediately and enjoy!
Nutrition:
Calories 195 Fat 12.2g Carbohydrates 8.1g Protein 6.9g

81.   Crispy Breaded Tofu Nuggets

Preparation Time: 10 minutes
Cooking time: 15 minutes
Servings: 4
Ingredients:
1 block extra firm tofu
1 cup panko breadcrumbs
2 flax eggs let sit 5 minutes before using
½ cup vegetable broth
1 tablespoon lite soy sauce
½ cup all-purpose flour
1 ½ teaspoons paprika
½ teaspoon onion powder
½ teaspoon garlic powder
½ teaspoon cayenne pepper
¼ teaspoon salt
¼ teaspoon fresh ground black pepper
Directions:
Preheat oven to 400° F. Line a baking sheet with parchment paper.
Slice the tofu into 10 squares. Cut the tofu into 5 slices along the long edge, and then cut each column in half to make squares. Lightly press each slice of tofu with a paper towel to remove some of the liquid.
To make the marinade, stir together the vegetable broth and soy sauce in a shallow pan. Marinate the tofu in the vegetable broth mixture for at least 10 minutes.
Prepare 3 bowls: one with the flour, one with panko breadcrumbs and spices, and one with the flax eggs. Coat the tofu in the flour, then the flax eggs, and finally the panko
Bake at 400° F on the parchment-lined baking sheet for 15 minutes. Carefully flip the tofu bites over, and then bake for another 15 minutes. They're ready when golden brown and crispy. Enjoy!
Nutrition:
Calories 127
Fat 0
Carbohydrates 23g
Protein 5g

82.   Rosemary Toasted Walnuts

Preparation Time: 10 minutes
Cooking time: 10-15 minutes
Servings: 8
Ingredients
2 cups raw walnuts
2 tablespoons fresh rosemary, finely chopped
¼ cup olive oil
½ teaspoon salt
1 teaspoon pepper
Directions:
Preheat oven to 350° F. Line a baking sheet with parchment paper.
In a bowl, whisk together olive oil, rosemary, salt, and pepper.
Add in walnuts and toss until completely covered in olive oil mixture.
Bake the walnuts for 10-15 minutes in the oven, tossing every 4-5 minutes until their golden brown. The walnuts cook quickly, so be careful not to burn them. Enjoy!
Nutrition:
Calories 223
 Fat 23g
Carbohydrates 5g
Protein 4g

83.   Cream Cheese Stuffed Celery

Preparation Time: 10 minutes
Cooking time: 10 minutes
Servings: 12
Ingredients
10 stalks celery, rinsed and dried well
16 oz. (2 packages) cream cheese, softened to room temperature
1 tablespoon milk
1 ¼ oz. (1 packet) vegetable soup mix
½ cup walnut chips
½ cup bacon pieces, for topping
Directions:
Cut dried celery stalks into 3 each. Set aside.
In a bowl, using an electric mixer, combine cream cheese and milk. Add dry vegetable soup mix and stir well.
Stuff celery with cream cheese mixture. If your mixture is thin enough, you can use a piping bag with tip and pipe the stuffing into the celery.
Sprinkle with walnut chips or bacon pieces (optional). Enjoy!
Nutrition:
Calories: 208
Fat: 18g
Carbohydrates: 9g
Protein:5g

CHAPTER 11:

Sirtfood Diet Soup Recipes

84.   Celery, Curry and Quinoa Soup

Preparation Time: 10 minutes
Cooking time: 10 minutes
Servings: 4
Ingredients:
1 cup. celery
8 tbsp. unsalted cashew nuts
Salt to taste
Curry to taste
Chili pepper Q.B.
8 tbsp. of quinoa
Directions:
Peel and cut the carrots into cubes, cook them in 700 ml of water until cooked. In the meantime, wash the quinoa and boil it in boiling, salted water for the time provided on the package.
Once the celery is cooked, blend it, and add the chopped cashews, curry, chili pepper to taste, and salt. Drain the quinoa and combine it with the rest. If the soup should turn out to be too liquid, cook it for a few more minutes until it is more compact.
Nutrition:
Calories 209.3
Fat 6.9g
Carbohydrates 31.4g
Protein 6.9g

85. Cabbage Soup

Preparation Time: 10 minutes
Cooking time: 15 minutes
Servings: 4
Ingredients
 1 cup black cabbage leaves
 1 leek
 4 or more slices of bread - 2-3 small carrots 1
Onion
1 potato - 2-3 celery ribs
Salt, pepper
Coriander seeds
2 tbsp. Almond flour
2 tbsp. baking powder
2 tbsp. EVO oil
Directions:
Wash and clean the vegetables. Prepare the broth with about 1 liter of slightly salted water and the carrots, onion, potato, and celery. Brown the leek cut into rings in oil and then adds the cabbage cut into strips 5-10 mm thick. Add salt and pepper and sprinkle with plenty of ground coriander. Let it season for a few minutes. When the cabbage begins to wither, add the stock, keeping about one glass aside, and leave to cook over low heat for 10-15 minutes. In the meantime, blend the potato with the stock set aside to add it to the cabbage 5 minutes before the end of cooking. Toasting slices of bread. Mix the almond flour with the baking powder and a pinch of salt to obtain a sort of 'grana.' When the cabbage is ready, in a bowl place cabbage in layers in broth, bread, and 'grana' until exhausted (if available for the last layer, you can add breadcrumbs to flour and yeast). Sprinkle with a drizzle of oil and bake in a preheated oven for half an hour (or until grating is satisfactory). Notes the cabbage ribs are not to be eliminated: they give the soup a crunchy note. An excellent solution to serve would be to cook directly in single-serving bowls. You can also do it with Savoy cabbage. For now, teetotalers: Red from Barbera grapes of Coli Piacentini, slightly sparkling, 15∘C 3,224
Nutrition:
Calories 85 Fat 0.6g Carbohydrates: 21g
Protein 4.2 g

86. Chickpea, Potato and Porcini Soup

Preparation Time: 10 minutes
Cooking time: 5 minutes
Servings: 4
Ingredients
5 small potatoes
 1 carrot 1
Courgette 1
Or 2 small washers of leek 1 tuft
Of parsley 1
L and 1/2 water
1 pack of canned chickpeas
1 or 2 porcini mushrooms 1
Sprig of rosemary
1 splash of red wine
 To taste

Directions:
Peel the potatoes, carrot, zucchini, leek, and boil them with a tuft of parsley together with water. In the meantime, fry the rosemary needles in a pan for a minute, to which you will add the professionally cleaned and diced porcini mushrooms. Skip them for a few minutes and add a splash of white wine; have the wine removed, and if they are too dry, add a ladle of broth; cook them covered. After about 30 minutes, remove all the vegetables from the broth except 3 potatoes; add 3/4 of the box of chickpeas and blend with the mini primer. Add salt and add the whole chickpeas, the other 2 potatoes cut into cubes and the cooked mushrooms. Cook for another 5 minutes so that the ingredients mix well and... Ready! If you like, you can add cubes of toasted bread in the oven.

Nutrition:
Calories 310
Fat 65 g
Carbohydrates: 31g
Protein 10 g
Cholesterol: 15mg

87.　　　Onion Soup

Preparation Time: 15 minutes
Servings: 4
Ingredients
 4 tbsp. white onions
 5 cups of vegetable stock
 Half a glass of water
 2 tbsp. of flour
 Some sage leaves
 Salt and pepper
 Evo oil
 Slices of homemade bread
 Aromatic vegetable cheese or yeast flakes
Directions:
Peel the onions, wash them, and cut them into very thin slices, put them on the fire with a drizzle of oil, and half a glass of water. Cook covered for 15 minutes, adding a few sage leaves; salt, pepper. Add 2 tablespoons of flour to the stewed onions, stir to mix well, add the boiling stock, cover, and cook over low heat for 50 minutes. Put the slices of toasted bread on the bottom of the bowls, sprinkle them with grated vegetable cheese with the large hole grater, or yeast in flakes, pour the onion soup, adding a sprinkling of pepper to taste.
Nutrition:
Calories: 290
Fat: 9.6 g
Carbohydrates: 33.4g
Protein 16.8 g

88.   Onion Soup 2

Preparation Time: 10 minutes
Cooking time: 50-60 minutes
Servings: 2
Ingredients
2 cups blonde onions
1 tsp. of flour
5 cups of vegetable stock
Laurel
Thyme
Sage
Olive oil
Directions:
Cut the onions into thin slices. Fry them in a high-sided saucepan with oil and 2 tablespoons of water. Continue cooking for 10 minutes. After this time, add the chopped aromatic herbs, season, and sprinkle with flour, mixing it. Once absorbed, add the stock, and continue cooking for 50-60 minutes, depending on whether you prefer a more liquid or more substantial soup. Notes Serve at will with scented Croutons or Croutons with sage.
Nutrition:
Calories: 290
Fat: 9.6 g
Carbohydrates: 33.4g
Protein 16.8 g

89.   Tomato Soup

Preparation Time: 10 minutes
Cooking time: 5 minutes
Servings: 1
Ingredients
 A cup of tomato puree or pulp
 A handful of thawed or dried mushrooms
 A celery stalks
 3 borettane onions
 A handful of shots of your choice
 1 teaspoon of vegetable nut powder
Directions:
Add a little water to the sauce, the chopped onions, the chopped celery, the mushrooms, and the nut. Cook until it reaches gravy consistency. Before serving, add the sprouts.
Nutrition:
Calories: 217
Fat: 8.3 g
Carbohydrates: 33.6g
Protein 7.1 g

90.   Celery Soup

Preparation Time: 10 minutes
Cooking time: 10 minutes
Servings: 6
Ingredients
10 medium potatoes
1 celery stalk
1 tablespoon of the organic granulated vegetable nut without salt
Water to cover the whole (about two liters)
Integral sea salt at will
Pepper
Directions:
Peel the potatoes cut them into chunks and put them in a pressure cooker; add the celery cut into pieces, of which only the tender inner part and a few leaves will be used. Add water until everything is well covered, add the cube, and at will some whole sea salt. Close the pot, and when it starts whistling, lowers the flame, cooking for 10 minutes. Turn it off, let the pressure run out, open, and add a little pepper. It can be consumed in this way or, even better, with the mini primer blend directly into the pot to obtain a cream.
Nutrition:
Calories: 273
Fat: 16 g
Carbohydrates: 21g
Protein 12 g

91.   Asparagus Au Gratin

Preparation Time: 10 minutes
Cooking time: 5 minutes
Servings: 2
Ingredients
2 cups of asparagus,
Vegan cheese Vegourmet Santeciano or a brick of Tofumargarina
olive oil
Salt
Directions:
Wash the asparagus after removing the hardest part of the stem. Steam them for 5 minutes, put them in an ovenproof dish greased with margarine or oil, sprinkle them with grated Santeciano Vegourmet Santeciano cheese with the large hole grater, or the Tofu cake (better a Silk Tofu that remains in small pieces like grated cheese) and let gratin in the oven already hot for a few minutes.
Nutrition:
Calories: 123.2
Fat: 7.2g
Carbohydrates: 4.0g
Protein 12 g

CHAPTER 12:

Sirtfood Diet Coffee Recipes

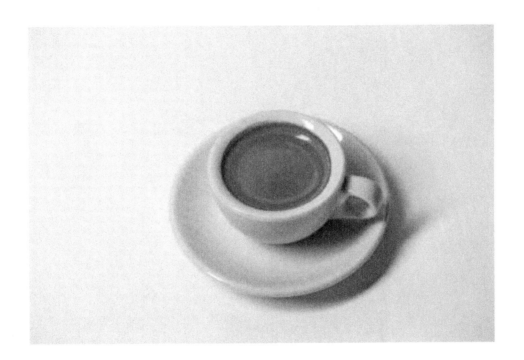

92.   Cappuccino Sauce

Preparation Time: 10 minutes
Servings: 2
Ingredients:
2 Express, short servings
1 Cup of milk
Directions:
Pour the milk into a saucepan

Put the espresso maker's steam nozzle a third of the way into the pitcher to make the milk foamy and open the steam valve all the way.

Do not let the milk boil or get too hot. Put the thermometer for the candy into the pitcher. Heat the milk to 175 degrees F. Evite heating the milk too hot. Close the Valve for steam.

Have espresso packed. Pour into serving cups until roughly a quarter of the cup is filled with coffee.

Stir the milk into the serving cups before pouring in. If you've poured much of the milk into the coffee, place a spoon under the milk, you're pouring on top of the coffee to create a coating of foamy milk.

Willing to serve.

Nutrition:

Calories: 80

Protein 15g

Fiber 3g

93.   Recipe by Granita

Preparation Time: 10 minutes
Servings: 1
Ingredients:
6 Espresso servings, at room temperature, short
3 Spoonful of sugar
16 Cubble of ice
2 Cups hot water
Directions:
Pour espresso in a blender. Stir in the water.
Add 90 seconds of sugar and espresso together. Stop the Mixer.
Add ice and water to taste. Mix in until smooth.
Pour into cups to serve.
Willing to serve.
Nutrition:
Calories: 202.5
Carbohydrate: 33.3g
Protein 8.1g
Fat: 4.8g

94.   Greek "Ouzo" Formula Coffee

Preparation Time: 1 minute
Servings: 1
Ingredients
2 Greek coffee tablecloths
2 Sugar Teaspoons
1 "ouzo" teaspoon (typical Greek alcohol)
Water: 2 *; 3 oz. cups
Directions:
Add the Ouzo inside after you have prepared your coffee and serve.
Nutrition:
Calories: 101
Fat: 0
Carbohydrates: 0g
Protein 0

95. Turkish coffee Recipe with "Fennel Seeds"
Preparation Time: 1 minute
Servings: 1
Directions:

Same as the above recipe, but instead of cardamom, you must use fennel seeds.
So, go ahead and enjoy great coffee!
Nutrition:
Calories: 202.5
Carbohydrate: 33.3g
Protein 8.1g
Fat: 4.8g

96. Classical Spanish Recipe for Coffee

Preparation Time: 1 minute
Servings: 1
Ingredients:
Appropriate for one human (High glass)
4 cups of Spanish coffee syrup
1 Bio espresso shot
0.75 teaspoons of low-fat steamed milk
Directions:
Take the blender cup clean and empty; pour all your ingredients into the cup. Mix it for a bit, before it mixes equally.
Upon completion, take a large empty bottle and pour the hot coffee into the container.
Finally, now you can enjoy your Spanish Coffee.
Nutrition:
Calories: 27
Carbohydrate: 6g
Protein 1g
Fat: 0.2

97.   Spanish and Latte Coffee Recipes

Preparation Time: 1 minutes
Servings: 1
Ingredients:
Spanish coffee syrup and chocolate syrup two tablespoons, respectively
1 Vegan espresso shot
0.75 Cup of steamed low-fat milk
5 to 8 cubes of ice
Some whipped cream (optional: you can put some whipped cream if you like it)
Directions:
Take one blender cup and put all the ingredients into the cup except whipped cream, which will be using.
if you like cold coffee, you can now put some ice cubes before you blend it.
Blend it with low speed until all well mixed.
Take an empty glass to pour your latte into the glass.
Finally, if you like whipped cream, put it on top of the latte before you serve it.
Nutrition:
Calories: 124
Carbohydrate: 15g
Protein 3g
Fat: 5g

98. Low Sugar Peaches and Spice Latte Recipe

Preparation Time:1 minute
Servings: 1
Ingredients
Enough for one person
2 tablespoons of peach with low sugar and cinnamon syrup respectively
1 Bio espresso shot
0.75 tablespoons of low-fat steamed milk
3 or 4 cubes of ice
1 small spoonful of cinnamon powder as a garnish to use at the last stage
Directions:
Put together all the ingredients in the blender cup except garnish, which we will use.
Blend it with medium speed for 1 minute until they are well mixed.
Take an empty glass to pour your latte into the glass.
At last, spread the powder of cinnamon top of the latte before you serve your latte.
Nutrition:
Calories: 80
Carbohydrate: 20g
Protein 0
Fat:0

CHAPTER 13:

Sirtfood Diet Recipes around the World

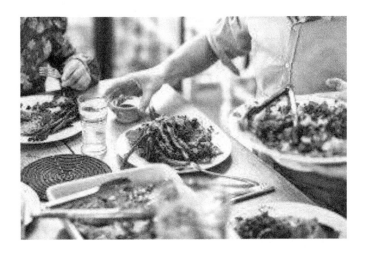

99. Turmeric Extract Poultry & Kale Salad with Honey Lime Dressing

Preparation Time: 10 minutes
Cooking time: 30 minutes
Servings: 2
Ingredients:
For the chicken:
1 teaspoon coconut oil
1/2 tool brown onion, diced
250-300 g/ 9 oz. hens mince or diced up her thighs
1 large garlic clove, finely diced
1 tsp turmeric powder
1teaspoon lime passion

Juice of 1/2 lime
1/2 tsp salt + pepper
For the salad:
6 broccoli stalks or broccoli florets
2 tablespoons pumpkin seeds (pepitas).
3 huge kale leaves, stems eliminated and chopped.
1/2 avocado, sliced.
Handful of fresh coriander leaves, chopped.
Handful of fresh parsley leaves, sliced.
For the clothing:
3 tablespoons lime juice.
1 small garlic clove, finely grated.
3 tbsps. Extra-virgin olive oil (I made use of 1 tbsp. avocado oil and * 2 tbsps. EVO).
1 tsp raw honey.
1/2 tsp wholegrain or Dijon mustard.
1/2 teaspoon sea salt and pepper.
Directions:
Warm the ghee or coconut oil in a small frying pan over medium-high warmth. Include the onion and sauté on medium heat for 4-5 mins, until golden. Include the hen dice as well as garlic and mix for 2-3 minutes over medium-high warm, breaking it apart.
Add the turmeric extract, lime enthusiasm, lime juice, salt, and pepper, and cook, frequently mixing, for a further 3-4 mins. Establish the cooked dice apart.
While the poultry is cooking, bring a small saucepan of water to steam. Add the broccolini and prepare for 2 mins. Wash under cold water as well as cut into 3-4 pieces each.
Include the pumpkin seeds to the frying pan from the poultry and toast over tool warmth for 2 mins, often mixing to avoid burning season with a little salt. Allot. Raw pumpkin seeds are too high to make use of.
The area sliced Kale in a salad bowl as well as pour over the clothing. Utilizing your hands, throw as well as massage the Kale with the dress. This will undoubtedly soften the Kale, kind of like what citrus juice does to fish or beef carpaccio-- it 'cooks' it slightly.
Finally toss via the prepared hen, broccolini, fresh, natural herbs, pumpkin seeds, and avocado pieces.
Nutrition:
Calories: 368 Carbohydrate: 30.3g Protein 6.7g Fat: 27.6g

100. Buckwheat Pasta with Chicken Kale & Miso Dressing

Preparation Time:15 minutes
Cooking time: 15 minutes
Servings: 2
Ingredients:
For the noodles:
2-3 handfuls of kale leaves (eliminated from the stem as well as approximately cut).
150 g/ 5 oz. 100% buckwheat noodles.
3-4 shiitake mushrooms cut.
1 tsp coconut oil or ghee.
1 brownish onion carefully diced.
1 medium free-range chicken breast cut or diced.
1 long red chili very finely sliced (seeds in or out depending upon how warm you like it).
2 big garlic cloves finely diced.
2-3 tablespoons Tamari sauce (gluten-free soy sauce).
For the miso dressing:
1 1/2 tbsp. fresh, natural miso.
1 tbsp. Tamari sauce.
1 tbsp. extra-virgin olive oil.
1 tbsp. lemon or lime juice.
1 teaspoon sesame oil (optional).
Directions:
Bring a tool saucepan of water to steam. Include the Kale as well as cook for 1 min, up until a little wilted. Remove as well as reserve yet schedule the water and bring it back to the boil. Add the soba noodles and chef according to the bundle guidelines (typically about 5 mins). Rinse under cold water and allotted.
Then pan fry the mushrooms in coconut oil (concerning a tsp) for 2-3 minutes until gently browned on each side. Sprinkle with sea salt and allotted.
In the very same frypan, warmth a lot more coconut oil or ghee over medium-high warm. Sauté onion and chili for 2-3 mins and then add the poultry pieces. Cook 5 mins over medium warmth, stirring a couple of times,

after that, add the garlic, tamari sauce, and a little splash of water. Cook for a more 2-3 mins, often mixing till hen is cooked via.

Lastly, include the kale and soba noodles and toss with the poultry to warm up.

Mix the dressing and drizzle over the noodles right at the end of cooking; this way, you will certainly maintain all those beneficial probiotics in the miso to life as well as energetic.

Nutrition:

Calories: 260

Carbohydrate: 35.3g

Protein 15g

Cholesterol: 50g

Fat: 27.6g

101. Asian King Shellfish Stir-Fry with Buckwheat Noodles

Preparation Time:10 minutes
Cooking time: 10 minutes
Servings: 4
Ingredients:
150g shelled raw king shellfishes, deveined.
2 tsp tamari (you can make use of soy sauce if you are not preventing gluten).
2 tsp extra virgin olive oil.
75g soba (buckwheat noodles).
One garlic clove finely sliced.
One bird's eye chili finely chopped.
1 tsp finely sliced fresh ginger.
20g red onions, sliced.
40g celery, trimmed, and cut.
75g environment-friendly beans, chopped.
50g kale approximately sliced.
100ml poultry stock.
5g Lovage or celery leaves
Directions:
Warm a frying pan over a high warm, then prepare the prawns in 1 tbsp. of the tamari as well as one teaspoon of the oil for 2-- 3 mins. Transfer the prawns to a small round plate. Wipe the pan out, as you're more likely to use it again.
Cook the noodles in boiling water for 5-- 8 minutes or as routed on the package. Drainpipes and allot.
At the same time, fry the garlic, chili and ginger, red onion, celery, beans, and Kale in the continuing to be oil over a tool-- high heat for 2-- 3 mins. Include the supply as well as offer the boil, then simmer momentarily or more, till the veggies are prepared however still crunchy.
Include the shellfishes, noodles, and Lovage/celery leaves to the frying pan, bring back to the boil, then eliminate from the warm and offer.
Nutrition:
Calories: 311 Carbohydrate: 52.7g Protein 26.7g
Cholesterol: 165g
Fat: 2.7g

102.   Aromatic Chicken Breast with Kale and Red Onions and a Tomato and Chili Salsa

Preparation Time:10 minutes
Cooking time: 20 minutes
Servings: 1
Ingredients:
4oz. skinless, boneless chicken breast
2 teaspoons ground turmeric - juice of 1/4 lemon
.5oz. extra virgin olive oil - 2oz. kale, chopped
.70oz. red onion, sliced
1 teaspoon chopped fresh ginger - 2oz. buckwheat
For the salsa
1 medium tomato
1 Thai chili, finely chopped
.5oz. capers, finely chopped
1oz. parsley, finely chopped
juice of 1/4 lemon
Directions:
To make the salsa, remove the eye from the tomato and chop it very finely, taking care to keep as much of the liquid as possible. Mix with the chili, capers, parsley, and lemon juice. You could put everything in a blender, but the end result is a little different.
Heat the oven to 425ºF (220ºC). Marinate the chicken breast in 1 teaspoon of the turmeric, the lemon juice, and a little oil. Leave for 5 to 10 minutes.
Heat an ovenproof frying pan until hot, then add the marinated chicken and cook for a minute or so on each side, until pale golden, then transfer to the oven (place on a baking tray if your pan isn't ovenproof) for 8 to 10 minutes or until cooked through. Remove from the oven, cover with foil, and leave to rest for 5 minutes before serving.
Meanwhile, cook the kale in a steamer for 5 minutes. Fry the red onions and the ginger in a little oil, until soft but not browned, then add the cooked kale and fry for another minute.
Cook the buckwheat according to the package instructions with the remaining teaspoon of turmeric. Serve alongside the chicken, vegetables, and salsa.
Nutrition:
Calories: 300g Carbs: 16g Fat: 13g Protein: 30g

103.   Baked Salmon Salad with Creamy Mint Dressing-Sirt Food Recipes

Preparation Time:5 minutes
Cooking time: 20 minutes
Servings: 1
Ingredients:
One salmon fillet
2 tbsp. blended salad leaves.
2 tbsp. young spinach leaves.
Two radishes cut and thinly sliced.
5cm item cucumber, cut into chunks.
Two spring onions trimmed as well as sliced.
One little handful parsley roughly sliced.
For the dressing:
1 tsp low-fat mayonnaise.
0.5oz. natural yogurt.
0.5oz. rice vinegar.
Two leaves mint carefully cut.
Salt as well as freshly ground
Directions:
Preheat the oven to 180 or 200 ° C
Place the salmon on a cooking tray and cook for 16-- 18 mins till just cooked via. Remove from the oven and set aside. The salmon is equally lovely hot, or cold in the salad. Simply cook skin side down of salmon and get rid of the salmon from the surface utilizing a fish slice after cooking. It must slide off quickly when cooked.
In a small dish, mix the mayo, yogurt, rice wine vinegar, mint leaves, as well as salt and pepper with each other and leave to represent at the very least 5 minutes to allow the.
Tastes to establish.
Organize the salad leaves and spinach on a serving plate and top with the radishes, cucumber, spring onions as well as parsley. Flake the prepared salmon onto the salad and drizzle the clothing over.
Nutrition:
Calories: 340 Carbohydrate: 7g
Protein 26.7g Cholesterol: 15g Fat: 2.7g

104.   Choc Chip Granola

Preparation Time:5 minutes
Cooking time: 20 minutes
Servings:
Ingredients:
1 cup high oats.
4 tbsp. pecans, about. Sliced.
3 tbsp. light olive oil.
1 tbsp. butter.
1 tbsp. dark brown sugar.
2 tbsp. rice malt syrup.
Dark delicious chocolate chips.
Directions:
Preheat your oven to 160 or 180 ° C. Line a big cooking tray with a silicone sheet or cooking parchment.

Mix the oats and pecans in a large dish. In a small non-stick frying pan, delicately heat the olive oil, butter, brownish sugar, and rice malt syrup until the butter has melted as well as the sugar and even syrup have liquefied. Do not permit to boil. Put the syrup over the oats and stir extensively until the oats are covered.

Disperse the granola over the cooking tray, spreading right into the corners. Leave clumps of mix with spacing as opposed to an even spread out. Cook in the stove for 20 minutes till just tinged gold brownish at the edges. Get rid of the furnace and entrust to cool on the tray entirely.

When high, break up any larger swellings on the tray with your fingers and then mix in the delicious chocolate chips. Scoop the granola into an airtight tub or container. The granola will maintain for at least two weeks.
Nutrition:
Calories: 220
Carbohydrate: 35g
Fat: 6g
Protein: 8g

105.   Fragrant Asian Hotpot-Sirt Food

Preparation Time:10 minutes
Cooking time: 10 minutes
Servings: 4
Ingredients:

1 tsp tomato purée.
One-star anise crushed (or 1/4 tsp ground anise).
Little handful parsley, stalks carefully sliced.
Little handful coriander, stalks finely cut.
Juice of 1/2 lime.
2 cups chicken supply, fresh or made with one dice.
1/2 carrot.
4 tbsp. broccoli, cut into tiny florets.
4 tbsp.. beansprouts.
raw tiger prawns.
firm tofu, sliced.
4 tbsp. rice noodles, cooked according to package guidelines.
4 tbsp. cooked water chestnuts, drained pipes.
1 tbsp. sushi ginger, sliced.
1 tbsp. good-quality miso paste.

Directions:
Place the tomato purée, celebrity anise, parsley stalks, coriander stalks, lime juice, and poultry supply in a huge pan and bring to a simmer for 10 minutes.
Add the carrot, broccoli, shellfishes, tofu, noodles as well as water chestnuts and simmer delicately until the shellfishes are prepared through. Remove from the warm and mix in the sushi ginger and even miso paste.
Serve sprayed with the parsley as well as coriander leaves.

Nutrition:
Calories: 1077
Carbohydrate: 73g
Fat: 47g
Protein:79g

CHAPTER 14:

Sirtfood Diet Raw Desserts

106. Raw Vegan Walnuts Pie Crust & Raw Brownies

Preparation Time:10 minutes
Cooking time: 10 minutes
Servings: 4
Ingredients
1 1/2 cups walnuts
1 cup pitted dates
1 1/2 tsp. Ground vanilla beans
1/3 cup unsweetened Cocoa powder
Topping for raw Brownies:
1/3 cup walnut butter
Directions:
Add walnuts to a Food processor or blender. Mix until finely ground.
Add the vanilla, dates, and Cocoa powder to the blender. Mix well and optionally add a couple drops of water at a time to make the mixture stick together.
This is a basic Raw Walnuts Pie Crust recipe.
If you need Pie Crust than spread it thinly in a 9 inch disc and add filling.
If you want to make raw Brownies, then transfer the mixture into a small dish and top with walnut butter.
Nutrition:
Calories: 214.5
Carbohydrate: 7.1g
Fat: 20.1g
Protein: 5.4g

107.   Raw Vegan Reese's Sirt Cups

Preparation Time:5 minutes
Cooking time: 10 minutes
Servings: 4
 Ingredients:

"Peanuts" Butter Filling
1 cup walnut butter
2 Tbsp. pitted dates
2 Tbsp. melted coconut oil
Superfoods Chocolate Part:
1/2 cup cacao powder
3 Tbsp. pitted dates
1/3 cup coconut oil (melted)
Directions:
Mix the "Peanut" butter filling Ingredients. Put a spoonful of the mixture into each muffin cup.
Refrigerate. Mix Superfoods Chocolate Ingredients. Put a spoonful of the Superfoods Chocolate mixture over the "Peanut" butter mixture. Freeze!
Nutrition:
Calories: 240
Carbohydrate: 26g
Fat: 12g
Protein: 6g

108.   Strawberry Frozen Yoghurt

Preparation Time:2 Hours
Servings: 4
Ingredients
450g (1lb) plain yoghurt 175g (6oz) strawberries Juice of 1 orange
1 tablespoon honey
Directions:
Place the strawberries and orange Juice into a Food processor or blender and blitz until smooth. Press the mixture through a serve into a large bowl to remove seeds. Stir in the honey and yoghurt. Transfer the mixture to an ice-cream maker and follow the manufacturer's instructions. Alternative pour the mixture into a container and Place in the fridge for 1 hour. Use a fork to whisk it and break up ice crystals and Freeze for 2 hours.

Nutrition:
Calories: 149 Carbohydrate: 11.g Fat: 8g Protein: 8.5g

109.   Chocolate Brownies

Preparation Time:10 minutes
Cooking time: 30 minutes
Servings: 4
Ingredients
200g (7oz) dark Chocolate (min 85% Cocoa) 200g (70z) medjool dates, stone removed 100g (3½oz) walnuts, chopped
3 eggs
25mls (1fl oz.) melted coconut oil 2 teaspoons vanilla essence
½ teaspoon baking soda
Directions:
Place the dates, Chocolate, eggs, coconut oil, baking soda and vanilla essence into a Food processor and mix until smooth. Stir the walnuts into the mixture. Pour the mixture into a shallow baking tray. Transfer to the oven and bake at 180C/350F for 25-30 minutes. Allow it to cool. Cut into pieces and serve.
Nutrition:
Calories: 604 Carbohydrate: 46.36g Fat: 46.6g Protein: 0

110.   Crème Brûlée

Preparation Time:3 minutes
Servings: 4
Ingredients
400g (14oz) strawberries
300g (11oz) plain low fat yoghurt 125g (4oz) Greek yoghurt
100g (3½oz) brown sugar 1 teaspoon vanilla extract
Directions:
Divide the strawberries between 4 ramekin dishes. In a bowl combined the plain yoghurt with the vanilla extract. Spoon the mixture onto the strawberries. Scoop the Greek yoghurt on top. Sprinkle the sugar into each ramekin dish, completely covering the top. Place the dishes under a hot grill (broiler) for around 3 minutes or until the sugar has caramelised.
Nutrition:
Calories: 182 Carbohydrate: 0
Fat: 0 Protein: 0

111.   Pistachio Fudge

Preparation Time: 10 minutes
Servings: 4
Ingredients
225g (8oz) medjool dates
100g (3½ oz.) pistachio nuts, shelled (or other nuts) 50g (2oz) desiccated (shredded) coconut
25g (1oz) oats
2 tablespoon water
Directions:
Place the dates, nuts, coconut, oats and water into a Food processor and processor until the Ingredients are well mixed. Remove the mixture and roll it to 2cm (1 inch) thick. Cut it into 10 pieces and serve.
Nutrition:
Calories: 170 Carbohydrate: 31.g
Fat: 5g Protein: 1g

112.   Spiced Poached Apples

Preparation Time: 15 minutes
Servings: 4
Ingredients
4 apples
2 tablespoons honey
4 star anise
2 cinnamon sticks 300mls (½ pint) green tea
Directions:
Place the honey and green tea into a saucepan and bring to the boil. Add the apples, star anise and cinnamon. Reduce the heat and simmer gently for 15 minutes. Serve the apples with a dollop of crème fraiche or Greek yoghurt.
Nutrition:
Calories: 52
Carbohydrate: 13.8.g
Fat: 0.2g
Protein: 0.3g

113.   Black Forest Smoothie

Preparation Time: 2 minutes
Servings: 2
Ingredients
100g (3½oz) frozen cherries 25g (1oz) Kale
1 medjool date
1 tablespoon Cocoa powder 2 teaspoons chia seeds
200mls (7fl oz.) milk or soya milk
Directions:
Place all the Ingredients into a blender and process until smooth and creamy.
Nutrition:
Calories: 308
Carbohydrate: 15.g
Fat: 0
Protein: 0

114.   Creamy Coffee Smoothie

Preparation Time:2 minutes
Servings: 4
Ingredients
1 banana
1 teaspoon chia seeds 1 teaspoon coffee
½ avocado
120mls (4fl oz.) water
Directions:
Place all the Ingredients into a Food processor or blender and blitz until smooth. You can add a little crushed ice too. This can also double as a breakfast Smoothie.
Nutrition:
Calories: 127
Carbohydrate: 21g
Fat: 3g
Protein:5g

CHAPTER 15:

Phase 1 Recipes

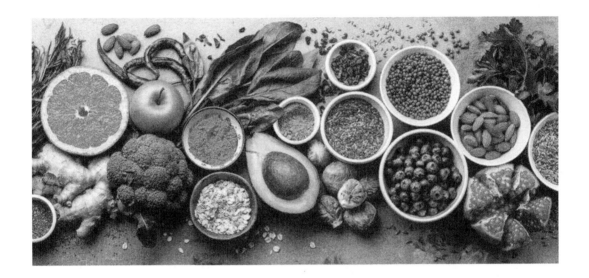

115.   Butternut Pumpkin with Buckwheat

Preparation Time: 10 minutes
Cooking time: 03 minutes
Servings: 4
 Ingredients
1 tbsp. of extra virgin olive oil
1 red onion, finely chopped
1 tbsp. fresh ginger, finely chopped
3 cloves of garlic, finely chopped
2 small chilies, finely chopped
1 tbsp. cumin
1 cinnamon stick

3 ½ cup turmeric
3 ½ cup chopped canned tomatoes
1 cup vegetable broth
8 tbsp. dates, seeded and chopped
One 2 tbsp. tin of chickpeas, drained
2 cups butter squash, peeled, seeded, and cut into pieces
buckwheat
1 tbsp. coriander, chopped
1 tbsp. parsley, chopped

Directions:

Preheat oven to 400 °.

Heat the olive oil in a frying pan and sauté the onion, ginger, garlic, and Thai chili. After two minutes, add cumin, cinnamon, and turmeric and cook for another two minutes while stirring.

Add the tomatoes, dates, stock, and chickpeas, stir well, and cook over low heat for 45 to 60 minutes. Add some water as required. In the meantime, mix the pumpkin pieces with olive oil and bake in the oven for about 30 minutes until soft.

Cook the buckwheat according to the Directions and add the remaining turmeric. When everything is cooked, add the pumpkin to the other ingredients in the roaster and serve with the buckwheat. Sprinkle with coriander and parsley.

Nutrition:

Calories: 82
Carbohydrate: 22g
Fat: 0g
Protein: 2g

116.   Chicken and Kale with Spicy Salsa

Preparation Time:10 minutes
Cooking time: 50 minutes
Servings: 1
Ingredients:
1 skinless, boneless chicken filet/breast
¼ cup buckwheat
1/4 lemon, juiced
1 tbsp. extra virgin olive oil
1 cup kale, chopped
1/2 red onion, sliced
1 tsp fresh ginger, chopped
2 tsp ground turmeric
Salsa:
1 tomato
3 sprigs of parsley, chopped
1 tbsp. chopped capers
1 chili, deseeded and minced use less if desired
Juice of 1/4 lemon
Directions:
Chop all ingredients above, just for the salsa, and set aside in a bowl.
Pre-eat the oven to 425 F.
Add a teaspoon of the turmeric, the lemon juice, and a little oil to the chicken, cover, and set aside for 10 minutes.
In a hot pan, slide the chicken and marinade and cook for 2-3 minutes each side, on high to sear it. Then, slide it all onto a baking-safe dish and cook for about 20 minutes or until cooked testing for pinkness).
Lightly steam the kale in a steamer, or on the stovetop with a lid and some water, for about 5 minutes. You want to wilt the kale, not boil, or burn it.
Sautee the red onions and ginger, and after 4-5 minutes, add the cooked kale and stir for 1 minute.
Cook the buckwheat, adding in the turmeric, see a package or look online if it was bought in bulk, for cooking Directions). Serve the chicken along with the buckwheat, kale, and spicy
Nutrition:
Calories: 590 Carbohydrate: 57g Fat: 18g Protein: 47g

117.   Smoked Salmon Sirt Salad

Preparation Time:10 minutes
Cooking time: 40 minutes
Servings: 4
Ingredients:
1 cup or ¼ packages if large of smoked salmon slices no cooking needed!
1 avocado, pitted, sliced, and scooped out
10 walnuts, chopped
5 Lovage or celery leaves), chopped
2 celery stalks, chopped or sliced thinly
½ small red onion, sliced thinly
1 Medjool pitted date, chopped
1 tbsp. capers
1 tbsp. extra virgin olive oil
1/4 of a lemon, juiced
5 sprigs of parsley, chopped
 Directions:
Wash and dry salad makings and vegetables, top with salmon.
Nutrition:
Calories: 100
Carbohydrate: 0g
Fat: 60g
Protein: 16g

118.   Tofu & Shiitake Mushroom Soup

Preparation Time: 10 minutes
Cooking time: 35 minutes
Servings: 4
Ingredients:

1 tbsp. dried wakame
1 tbsp. vegetable stock
1 cup shiitake mushrooms, sliced
1/3 cup miso paste
1* ½ cup. firm tofu, diced
2 green onion, trimmed and diagonally chopped
1 bird's eye chili, finely chopped

Directions:

Soak the wakame in lukewarm water for 10-15 minutes before draining.

In a medium-sized saucepan, add the vegetable stock and bring to the boil. Toss in the mushrooms and simmer for 2-3 minutes.

Mix miso paste with 3-4 tbsp of vegetable stock from the saucepan until the miso is entirely dissolved. Pour the miso-stock back into the pan and add the tofu, wakame, green onions, and chili, then serve immediately.

Nutrition:

Calories: 98
Carbohydrate: 7g
Fat: 4g
Protein: 8g

119.   Honey Chili Nuts

Preparation Time:10 minutes
Cooking time: 30 minutes
Servings: 4
Ingredients
150g 5oz walnuts
150g 5oz pecan nuts
50g 2oz softened butter
1 tablespoon honey
½ bird's-eye chili, very finely chopped and deseeded
126 calories per serving
Directions:
Preheat the oven to 180C/360F. Combine the butter, honey, and chili in a bowl, then add the nuts and stir them well. Spread the nuts onto a lined baking sheet and roast them in the oven for 10 minutes, stirring once halfway through. Remove from the oven and allow them to cool before eating.
Nutrition:
Calories: 561
Carbohydrate: 23.7g
Fat: 47.7g
Protein: 8g

120. Pomegranate Guacamole

Preparation Time:10 minutes
Cooking time: 40 minutes
Servings: 4
Ingredients
Flesh of 2 ripe avocados
Seeds from 1 pomegranate
1 bird's-eye chili pepper, finely chopped
½ red onion, finely chopped
Juice of 1 lime
151 calories per serving
Directions:
Place the avocado, onion, chili, and lime juice into a blender and process until smooth. Stir in the pomegranate seeds. Chill before serving. Serve as a dip for chop vegetables.
Nutrition:
Calories: 122
Carbohydrate: 10.2
Fat: 9.6g
Protein: 1.6g

121.   Chicken curry with potatoes and kale

Preparation Time:10 minutes
Cooking time: 20 minutes
Servings: 4
Ingredients
chicken breast, cut into pieces - 4 tbsp. of extra virgin olive oil
2 tbsp.. turmeric - 2 red onions, sliced
2 red chilies, finely chopped - 3 cloves of garlic, finely chopped
1 tbsp. freshly chopped ginger - 1 tbsp. curry powder
1 tin of small tomatoes (400ml) - 1 cup chicken broth
½ cup coconut milk - 2 pieces cardamom
1 cinnamon stick
3 cups potatoes mainly waxy)
1 tbsp. parsley, chopped
¾ cup kale, chopped
1 tbsp. coriander, chopped
Directions:
Marinate the chicken in a teaspoon of olive oil and a tablespoon of turmeric for about 30 minutes. Then fry in a high frying pan at high heat for about 4 minutes. Remove from the pan and set aside.
Heat a tablespoon of oil in a pan with chili, garlic, onion, and ginger. Boil everything over medium heat and then add the curry powder and a tablespoon of turmeric and cook for another two minutes, stirring occasionally. Add tomatoes; cook for another two minutes until finally chicken stock, coconut milk, cardamom, and cinnamon stick are added. Cook for about 45 to 60 minutes and add some broth if necessary.
In the meantime, preheat the oven to 425 °. Peel and chop the potatoes. Bring water to the boil, add the potatoes with turmeric and cook for 5 minutes. Then pour off the water and let it evaporate for about 10 minutes. Spread olive oil together with the potatoes on a baking tray and bake in the oven for 30 minutes.
When the potatoes and curry are almost ready, add the coriander, kale, and chicken and cook for five minutes until the chicken is hot.
Add parsley to the potatoes and serve with the chicken curry.
Nutrition:
Calories: 166.3 Carbohydrate: 19g Fat: 5.6g Protein: 11.1g

122.   Tofu and Curry

Preparation Time: 10 minutes
Cooking time: 30 minutes
Servings: 4
Ingredients:
8 oz. dried lentils red preferably
1 Cup boiling water
1 cup frozen edamame soybeans
7 oz. 1/2 of most packages firm tofu, chopped into cubes
2 tomatoes, chopped
1 lime juices
5-6 kale leaves, stalks removed and torn
1 large onion, chopped
4 cloves garlic, peeled and grated
1 large chunk of ginger, grated
1/2 red chili pepper, deseeded useless if too much
1/2 tsp ground turmeric
1/4 tsp cayenne pepper
1 tsp paprika
1/2 tsp ground cumin
1 tsp salt
1 tbsp. olive oil
Directions:
Add the onion, sauté in the oil for few minutes, then add the chili, garlic, and ginger for a bit longer until wilted but not burned. Add the seasonings, then the lentils, and stir. Add in the boiling water and cook for 10 minutes. Simmer for up to 30 minutes longer, so it will be stew-like but not overly mushy. You should check the texture of the lentils halfway, though.
Add tomato, tofu, and edamame, then lime juice and kale—test for when the kale is tender, and then it is ready to serve.
Nutrition:
Calories: 219
Carbohydrate: 8.4g
Fat: 17g
Protein: 12.6g

123.   Garbanzo Kale Curry

Preparation Time: 10 minutes
Cooking time: 45 minutes
Servings: 8
4 cups dry garbanzo beans
Curry Paste, but go **Ingredients**   low on the heat
1 cup sliced tomato
2 cups kale leaves
1/2 cup coconut milk
Directions:
Put ingredients in the slow cooker. Cover, & cook on low for 7 to 9 hours.
Nutrition:
Calories: 160
Carbohydrate: 11g
Fat: 11g
Protein: 4g

124.   Kale & Shiitake Stew

Preparation Time: 10 minutes
Cooking time: 40 minutes
Servings: 8
Ingredients
3 garlic cloves, minced
2 cups chopped onions
1/2 cup olive oil
Salt & 1 Tsp. ground pepper to taste
4 cups vegetable broth
2 pounds dry shiitake mushrooms
Directions:
Put ingredients in the slow cooker. Cover, & cook on low for 3 to 4 hours.
Nutrition:
Calories: 285
Carbohydrate: 40.2g
Fat: 2.6g
Protein: 14.7g

125. Kale & Chicken Stew

Preparation Time: 5 minutes
Cooking time: 55 minutes
Servings: 4
Ingredients
1 cup sliced leeks
1 sliced carrot
1 cup chopped onions
Salt & 1 Tsp. ground pepper to taste
2 cups chicken broth
3 cups kale
4 pounds of chicken
Directions:
Put ingredients in the slow cooker. Cover, & cook on low for 7 to 9 hours.
Nutrition:
Calories: 266.6
Carbohydrate: 33.1g
Fat: 25.6g
Protein: 22.7g

126.   Mushroom & Tofu Scramble

Preparation Time: 5 minutes
Cooking time: 35 minutes
Servings: 1
Ingredients
tofu, extra firm
1 tsp ground turmeric
1 tsp mild curry powder
1 tbsp.. kale, roughly chopped
1 tsp extra virgin olive oil
1 tbsp. red onion, thinly sliced
4 tbsp. mushrooms, thinly sliced
1 tbsp. parsley, finely chopped
Directions:
Place 2 sheets of kitchen towel under and on top of the tofu then rest a considerable weight such as saucepan onto the tofu, to ensure it drains off the liquid.
Combine the curry powder, turmeric, and 1-2 tsp of water to form a paste. Using a steamer cook kale for 3-4 minutes.
In a skillet, warm oil over medium heat. Add the chili, mushrooms, and onion, cooking for several minutes or until brown and tender.
Break the tofu into small pieces and toss in the skillet. Coat with the spice paste and stir, ensuring everything becomes evenly coated. Cook for up to 5 minutes, or until the tofu has browned, then add the kale and fry for 2 more minutes. Garnish with parsley before serving.
Nutrition:
Calories: 171.8
Carbohydrate: 0
Fat: 0
Protein: 5.4

127.   Prawn & Chili Pak Choi

Preparation Time: 5 minutes
Cooking time: 35 minutes
Servings: 4
Ingredients
¾ cup brown rice
1 Pak choi
4 tbsp. chicken stock
2 tbsp. extra virgin olive oil
1 garlic clove, finely chopped
4 tbsp. red onion, finely chopped
½ bird's eye chili, finely chopped
1 tsp freshly grated ginger
1 cup shelled raw king prawns
1 tbsp. soy sauce
1 tsp five-spice
1 tbsp. freshly chopped flat-leaf parsley
A pinch of salt and pepper
Directions:
Bring a medium-sized saucepan of water to the boil and cook the brown rice for 25-30 minutes, or until softened.
Tear the Pak choi into pieces. Warm the chicken stock in a skillet over medium heat and toss in the Pak choi, cooking until the Pak choi has slightly wilted.
In another skillet, warm olive oil over high heat. Toss in the ginger, chili, red onions, and garlic frying for 2-3 minutes.
Throw in the pawns, five-spice and soy sauce and cook for 6-8 minutes, or until the cooked throughout. Drain the brown rice and add to the skillet, stirring and cooking for 2-3 minutes. Add the Pak choi, garnish with parsley and serve.
Nutrition:
Calories: 163
Carbohydrate: 8.8g
Fat: 6.3g
Protein:15g

CHAPTER 16:

Phase 2 Recipes

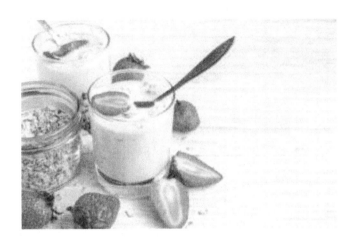

128.   Mango Smoothie

Preparation Time:5 minutes
Servings: 2
Ingredients
¼ cup with pieces of mango (40 gr) - ¼ cup shredded ripe avocado (56 gr)
½ cup ripe mango juice (125 ml) - ¼ cup vanilla yogurt (fat free) (50 gr)
1 tablespoon of lemon juice (15 ml) - 1 tablespoon of sugar (15 gr) Ice
cubes
Directions:
Take all the ingredients listed above and put them in the blender
Blend everything until you get a homogeneous mix- Serve in a large glass.
Add a little lemon juice and mix well. You can add pieces of mango at will.
Nutrition:
Calories: 240 Carbohydrate: 35g Fat: 7.8g Protein: 8.2g

129.   Blueberry Smoothie

Preparation Time: 3 minutes
 Servings: 2
Ingredients
A cup of skim milk (250 ml)
A cup of blueberries (140 gr)
A tablespoon of organic flaxseed oil (cold-pressed)
Directions:
Put the blueberries and milk in the blender
Blend for 2 or 3 minutes
Serve in a glass and add the flax seeds
Mix well.
Nutrition:
Calories: 162
Carbohydrate: 30g
Fat: 0.5g
Protein: 14g

130.   Peach Smoothie

Preparation Time: 3 minutes
Servings: 2
Ingredients
A cup of skim milk (250 ml)
A cup of peaches (150 gr)
Two tablespoons of organic flaxseed oil (cold-pressed)
Directions:
Put the peaches and milk in the blender
Blend for a few minutes
Serve in a glass and add the flax seeds
Mix well
Nutrition:
Calories: 300
Carbohydrate: 67.7g
Fat: 1.5g
Protein: 6g

131.   Pineapple Smoothie

Preparation Time: 3 minutes
Servings: 2
Ingredients
A cup of skim milk (250 ml)
Pineapple cut into pieces
A tablespoon of organic flaxseed oil
A few ices cube
Directions:
Put the pineapple and milk in the blender
Add the ice and blend for a few minutes
Pour the contents of the blender into a glass
Add the organic flaxseed oil
Mix well.
Nutrition:
Calories: 175 Carbohydrate: 37g Fat: 2.2g Protein: 4.4g

132.   Vegetable Smoothie

Preparation Time: 3 minutes
Servings: 4
Ingredients
½ cucumbers - ½ celery head - 2 cups of spinach (60 gr)
A handful of mint
3 carrots
½ handful of parsley
¼ pineapple, orange, and lemon
2 apples
Directions:
Place all the ingredients in the blender and mix until a homogeneous mix is obtained
Pour into a glass
For fast results, drink this smoothie regularly.
Nutrition:
Calories: 289 Carbohydrate: 58.6g Fat: 6.6g Protein: 5.9g

133. Natural Protein Shake

Preparation Time:3 minutes
Servings: 2
Ingredients
½ bananas - ½ cup of peanut butter (100 gr)
½ cup of fat-free milk (125 ml)
1 tablespoon of chocolate-flavored whey protein
From 6 to 8 ice cubes
Directions:
Pour all the ingredients into a blender
Blend for a few minutes until the mix becomes homogeneous and consistent
Pour the smoothie into a glass.
Nutrition:
Calories: 120 Carbohydrate: 9g Fat: 3 g Protein: 15 g

134. Hummus

Preparation Time:3 minutes
Servings: 2
Ingredients:
1 cup of boiled chickpea sauce
2 tbsp. tahina - 1 lemon
1 clove of garlic
1 teaspoon cumin seeds
4 tbsp. of oil - Salt
Paprika
Directions:
Remove the chickpeas peel, the cooking water (keep only a couple of spoons aside) and put them in a bowl.
Add the tahini sauce, cumin, garlic, lemon juice, and salt
Blend at maximum speed, gradually adding oil
If the hummus is too compact, add a couple of tablespoons of chickpea cooking water
Transfer the mixture to a bowl, sprinkle with paprika and serve the hummus
Nutrition:
Calories: 166 Carbohydrate: 14.3g Fat: 9.6 g Protein: 7.9 g

135.   Bacon Pancake

Preparation Time:3 minutes
Cooking time: 15 minutes
Servings: 12
Ingredients:
2 eggs
4 tbsp. of butter
1 cup of milk
1 cup of 00 flour
1 teaspoon salt
1 teaspoon of instant yeast
12 slices of bacon
Directions:
Separate the yolks from the whites beat the first with milk and melted butter and, separately, whip the latter with stiff peaks.
Add flour, salt and yeast to the milk mixture and mix, finally add the egg whites, stirring slowly and from the bottom up, so as not to disassemble them.
Brown 1 slice of bacon in a non-stick pan: when the edges start to brown, turn it over and pour a ladle of the mixture over it, so that while you gild the second side, you also cook the first side of the pancake.
When bubbles begin to form on the surface of the mixture, turn the pancake (with the bacon already incorporated) with a spatula and cook the second side as well.
Do this for all pancakes, stacking them on a plate as they are ready.
Bacon pancakes are ready: decorated as desired with maple syrup and serve.
Nutrition:
Calories: 420
Carbohydrate: 57g
Fat: 15 g
Protein: 15 g

136.   Stuffed Dried Cherry Tomatoes

Preparation Time: 5 minutes
Cooking time: 10 minutes
Servings: 4
Ingredients:
1 cup of dried tomatoes
1 cup of breadcrumbs
½ cup gr of grated pecorino cheese
1 clove of garlic
1 tbsp. of desalted capers
Extra virgin olive oil
Directions:
Chop bread, capers, and garlic and put them in a bowl together with the pecorino cheese and a drizzle of oil.
Mix until a crumbly but homogeneous mixture is obtained.
Spread the stuffing on half of each dried tomato, and then close the tomato as if to create a slightly open shell and fix the two halves with a toothpick.
Arrange all the tomatoes on a baking sheet without overlapping them and leaving the filling visible from the top.
Cook for 10 minutes in a preheated convection oven at 220 ° C (if necessary, turn on the grill in the last few minutes of cooking).
The stuffed dried cherry tomatoes are ready, serve them immediately.
Nutrition:
Calories: 5
Carbohydrate: 1.12.g
Fat: 0.06 g
Protein: 0.28 g

137.   Shrimp Canapé

Preparation Time: 5 minutes
Cooking time: 15 minutes
Servings: 4
Ingredients:
1 rolls of short crust pastry
Chives
Tarragon
1 cup of prawn tails
Butter
Salt
Brandy
1 lemon peel
1 cup of mayonnaise
Pink pepper
Directions:
Roll out the short crust pastry, sprinkle with a chopped aromatic herb to taste, then use a 7 cm pastry cutter to make the bases for your canapés and prick them.

Using an inverted (and lightly greased) muffin pan as a mold, give your molds the shape of exceedingly small tacos, taking care to leave the part with the herbs outside.

Bake for 10-15 minutes at 180 ° C in a preheated convection oven, then gently turn out and leave to cool.

In the meantime, season the prawn tails with salt and brandy and cook them in a pan with the butter.

Assemble the canapes: add 1 shrimp into each brisée base, and then decorate with mayonnaise, lemon peel, and pink pepper.

The prawn canapés are ready; you just must serve them and delight your guests.
Nutrition:
Calories: 180
Carbohydrate: 10g
Fat: 2 g
Protein: 12 g

138.   Cabbage Chips

Preparation Time: 10 minutes
Cooking time: 10 minutes
Servings: 2
Ingredients:
1 cup of black cabbage
6 tbsp. of extra virgin olive oil
1 tbsp. of flax seeds
1 tbsp. of sesame seeds
Salt
Pepper
Directions:
First, clean the cabbage, then dry the leaves with a cloth and remove the central rib.
Prepare the dressing in a bowl by mixing salt, pepper, oil, and seeds.
Arrange the leaves on the baking tray lined with parchment paper without overlapping them, and then sprinkle them with the dressing.
Then cook for 5-10 minutes, or until they are crunchy, at 180 ° C in a preheated oven.
The black cabbage chips are ready, serve them immediately, whole or chopped.
Nutrition:
Calories: 4
Carbohydrate: 1g
Fat: 0 g
Protein: 3 g

139. Savory Mushroom Muffins

Preparation Time: 10 minutes
Cooking time: 10 minutes
Servings: 8
Ingredients:
½ cup of 00 flour
2 tbsp. of parmesan
1/2 sachet of instant yeast for savory pies
1 cup of milk
1 egg
1 cup of mushrooms in oil
Salt
Pepper
Directions:
In a bowl, whisk the egg and milk, apart from mixing the flour, Parmesan and baking powder, salt, and pepper.
Add the flour and parmesan compote to the beaten egg and milk and mix everything with a wooden spoon.
Now add the mushrooms in oil to the dough (lift them with a fork from the jar so as not to add too much oil)
Stir quickly with a spoon so that the mushrooms are evenly distributed in the muffin dough
Pour the salted mushroom muffin mixture into buttered and floured muffin molds.
Turn on the oven at 180 degrees and cook for 20 minutes.
Leave to cool, and then serve your mushroom muffins.
Nutrition:
Calories: 182
Carbohydrate: 6g
Fat: 11 g
Protein: 10g

140.   Avocado Fries

Preparation Time: 10 minutes
Cooking time: 15 minutes
Servings: 4
Ingredients:
2 avocados
3 eggs
Rice flour
Breadcrumbs
1 lime
Cumin
Pepper
Salt
Seed oil
Directions:
Cut the avocado in half and remove the core and cut it into sticks. Then remove the peel
Beat the eggs with the salt, pepper, cumin, and grated lime zest.
Pass the avocado sticks first in the flour, then in the eggs and breadcrumbs. Then again in the eggs and breadcrumbs, thus obtaining a double breading.
Fry the avocado sticks in hot oil. When they are golden brown, drain, and place the fries obtained on a plate covered with paper towels.
Serve the avocado sticks immediately, accompanying them with the mayonnaise you have flavored with juice and lime peel.
Nutrition:
Calories: 131.9
Carbohydrate: 6.6g
Fat: 11.1 g
Protein: 4g

141.   Fruit Baskets

Preparation Time: 10 minutes
Cooking time: 20 minutes
Servings: 4
Ingredients
For the short crust pastry:
1 cup of 00 flour
1 egg
1 cup of icing sugar
1 cup of butter
Lemon peel
For the cream:
2 yolks
5oz. of sugar
88oz. of 00 flour
9oz.of milk
Vanilla bean
Lemon peel
To garnish:
1/2 kiwi
4oz. of strawberries
3oz. of blueberries
Mint
Directions:
Start preparing the pastry by adding flour, eggs, sugar, grated lemon peel, and chunks of butter. Work with your fingertips, starting from the center and gradually incorporating all the flour.

Once you have obtained homogeneous dough, wrap it in plastic wrap and leave it in the fridge for 30 minutes.

Once the dough is taken, roll it out on a floured work surface, obtaining a sheet of about 3mm.

With a pasta bowl, make circles and transfer them into the tart molds.

Prick the base with the prongs of a fork, and then cook the pastry shells in a preheated oven at 180 ° C for 15-20 minutes. Once ready, let it cool.

Now prepare the custard by adding the yolks and sugar.

Then add the flour and work until you get a cream.

Heat the milk with the vanilla stick and the lemon peel over the heat.

Before it reaches a boil, lift vanilla and lemon and transfer to the prepared mixture.

Stir and pass everything on the fire to thicken.

Pour the cream into a bowl, cover with the cling film and allow cooling completely.

Clean the fruit and cut it into small pieces.

Now fill the baskets of pastry with the cream, using a syringe for sweets.

Finally, garnish with the pieces of fruit and mint leaves.

Your fruit baskets are ready to be served.

Nutrition:

Calories: 100

Carbohydrate: 23g

Fat: 0 g

Protein:1g

CHAPTER 17:

The 6-Day Meal Plan

You can do This plan for up to two weeks, after which its all about adjusting it to suit your lifestyle. There are no set rules – just try to include as many Sirt foods as possible In your diet, which should make you feel healthier, more energetic and improve your skin, as well as making you leaner.

This super-healthy green Juice and these yummy choc balls are Sirtfood Diet staples.

All recipes serve one (unless otherwise started).

142. Sirtfood Bites

Preparation Time: 10 minutes
Cooking time: 10 minutes
Servings: 15-20 bites
Ingredients:
1 cup walnuts
2 tbsp. dark Chocolate (85% Cocoa solids), broken into pieces, or Cocoa nibs
1 cup Medjool dates, pitted
1 tbsp. Cocoa powder
1 tbsp. ground Turmeric
1 tbsp. extract virgin Olive oil
Scraped seeds of 1 vanilla pod or 1tsp vanilla extract
Directions:
Place the walnuts and Chocolate into a Food processor and blend until you Have a fine powder. Add all the other Ingredients and blend until the mixture forms a large ball. Add 2tbsp water to help bind it, if need.

Using your hands, make bite-sized balls from the mix and Refrigerate In an airtight container for at least 1-hour before serving. The balls will keep for up to a week In the fridge.
Nutrition:
Calories: 45
Carbohydrate: 7g
Fat: 1 g
Protein: 1g

Day 1
3 x Sirtfood green juices

2 x Sirtfood bites (you can substitute these for 15-20g of dark Chocolate if you wish)

1 x Sirtfood meal

143.   Asian King Prawn Stir-Fry

Preparation Time: 10 minutes
Cooking time: 10 minutes
Servings: 2
Ingredients:

¾ cup raw king prawn, shelled
2tsp tamari or soy sauce
2tsp extra virgin Olive oil
1 clove garlic, finely chopped
1 bird's eye chilli, finely chopped
1tsp fresh ginger, finely chopped
1 tbsp. red onions, sliced
2 tbsp. celery, trimmed and sliced
6 tbsp. green beans, chopped
4 tbsp. Kale, roughly chopped
1 cup chicken stock
¾ cup soba (buckwheat noodles)
1 tbsp. lovage or celery leaves

Directions:

In a frying plan over a high heat, cook the prawns In 1tsp tamari or soy sauce and 1tsp oil for 2-3 minutes. Transfer to a plate.

Add the remaining oil to the pan and fry the garlic, chilli, ginger, red onion, celery, beans and Kale over a medium-high heat for 2-3 minutes. Add the stock and bring to the boil, then simmer until the vegetables are cooked but still crunchy.

Cook the noodles In boiling water according to pack instructions. Drain and add the lovage or celery leaves, noodles and prawns to the pan. Bring back to the boil, then remove from the heat and serve.

Nutrition:

Calories: 100 Carbohydrate: 23g Fat: 0 g Protein: 1g

Day 2

3 x Sirtfood green juices

2 x Sirtfood bites

1 x Sirtfood meal

144.   Turkey Escalope

Preparation Time: 10 minutes
Cooking time: 10 minutes
Servings: 4
Ingredients:

1 cup cauliflower, roughly chopped
1 clove garlic, finely chopped
2 tbsp. red onion, finely chopped
1 bird's eye chilli, finely chopped
1tsp fresh ginger, finely chopped
2 tbsp. extra virgin Olive oil
2tsp ground Turmeric
2 tbsp. sun-dried tomatoes, finely chopped
1 tbsp. Parsley
1 cup turkey escalope
1tsp dried sage
Juice 1/2 lemon
1 tbsp. capers

Directions:

Place the cauliflower In a Food processor and pulse In 2-second burst to finely chop it until it resembles couscous. Sat aside. Fry the garlic, red onion, chilli and ginger In 1tsp of the oil until soft but not coloured. Add the Turmeric and cauliflower and cook for 1 minutes. Remove from the heat and add the sun-dried tomatoes and half the Parsley.

Coat the turkey escalope In the remaining oil and sage then fry for 5-6 minutes, turning regularly. When cooked, add the lemon Juice, remaining Parsley, capers and 1tbsp water to the pan to make a sauce, then serve.

Nutrition:

Calories: 117 Carbohydrate: 0g Fat: 2g Protein: 24g

Day 3

3 x Sirtfood green juices

2 x Sirtfood bites

1 x Sirtfood meal

145.   Aromatic Chicken

Preparation Time: 10 minutes
Cooking time: 10 minutes
Servings: 4
Ingredients:
For the salsa
1 large tomato - 1 bird's eye chilli, finely chopped
1 cup capers, finely chopped - 1 tbsp. Parsley, finely chopped
Juice 1/2 lemon
For the chicken
1 cup skinless, boneless chicken breast - 2tsp ground Turmeric
Juice 1/2 lemon - 1 cup extra virgin Olive oil - 2 tbsp. Kale, chopped
1 tbsp. red onion, sliced
1tsp fresh ginger, finely chopped
1 tbsp. buckwheat
Directions:
Heat the oven to 220ºC/200ºC fan/gas mark 7.
To make the salsa, finely chop the tomato, making sure you keep as much of the liquid as possible. Mix with the chilli, capers, Parsley and lemon Juice. Marinate the chicken breast In 1tsp of the Turmeric, lemon Juice and half the oil for 5-10 minutes.
Heat an ovenproof frying pan, add the marinated chicken and cook for a minutes on each side until golden, then transfer to the oven for 8-10 minutes or until cooked through. Remove, cover with foil and leave to rest for 5 minutes.
Cook the Kale In a steamer for 5 minutes. Fry the onion and ginger In the rest of the oil until soft but not coloured, then add the cooked Kale and fry for an other minutes.
Cook the buckwheat according to pack instructions with the remaining Turmeric, and serve.
Nutrition:
Calories: 439 Carbohydrate: 0g Fat: 0g Protein: 0g

Day 4
2 x Sirtfood green juices
 2 x Sirtfood meals

146.   Sirt Muesli

Preparation Time: 5 minutes
Servings: 4
Ingredients:

1 tbsp. buckwheat flakes
1 tsp. buckwheat puff
1 tbsp. coconut flakes or desiccated coconut
2 tbsp. Medjool dates, pitted and chopped
2 tbsp. walnuts, chopped
1 tbsp. Cocoa nibs
1 tbsp. strawberries, hulled and chopped
1 tbsp. plain Greek yoghurt (or vegan alternative, such as soya or coconut yoghurt)
Directions:
Mix all of the Ingredients together and serve (leaving out the strawberries and yoghurt if not serving straight away).

Nutrition:
Calories: 368
Carbohydrate: 54g
Fat: 16g
Protein: 26g

147. Pan-Fried Salmon Salad

Preparation Time: 10 minutes
Cooking time: 10 minutes
Servings: 2
Ingredients:
For the dressing
1 tbsp. Parsley
Juice 1/2 lemon
1 tbsp. capers
1 tbsp. extra virgin Olive oil
For the salad
1/2 avocado, peeled, stone and diced
1 cup cherry tomatoes, halved
1 tbsp. red onion, thinly sliced
2 tbsp. rocket
1 tsp. celery leaves
skinless salmon fillet
2tsp brown sugar
4 tbsp. chicory (head), halved lengthways
Directions:
Heat the oven to 220ºC/ 200ºC fan/gas mark 7.
To make the dressing, whizz the Parsley, lemon Juice, capers and 2tsp oil In a blender until smooth.
For the salad, mix the avocado, tomato, red onion, rocket and celery leaves together.
Rub the salmon with a little oil and sear it In an ovenproof frying pan for a minute. Transfer to a baking tray and cook In the oven for 5 minutes.
Mix the brown sugar with 1tsp oil and brush it over the Cut side of the chicory. Place cut-sides down In a hot frying pan and cook for 2-3 minutes, turning regularly. Dress the salad and serve together.
Nutrition:
Calories: 368 Carbohydrate: 54g
Fat: 16g Protein: 26g

Day 5
2 x Sirtfood green juices
2 x Sirtfood meals

148.   Strawberry Tabbouleh

Preparation Time:5 minutes
Servings: 2
Ingredients:

4 tbsp. buckwheat
1tbsp ground Turmeric
1 cup avocado
4 tbsp. tomato
1 tbsp. red onion
2 tbsp. Medjool dates, pitted
1 tbsp. capers
2 tbsp. Parsley
1 cup strawberries, hulled
1 cup extra virgin Olive oil
Juice 1/2 lemon
1 tbsp. rocket

Directions:
Cook the buckwheat with the Turmeric according to pack instructions. Drain and cool.

Finely chop the avocado, tomato, red onion, dates, capers and Parsley and mix with the cooked buckwheat.

Slice the strawberries and gently mix into the salad with the oil and lemon Juice. Serve on the rocket.

Nutrition:
Calories: 138g
30g Carbs: 30g
0g Fat: 0
Protein: 0

149.   Miso-Marinated Baked Cod

Preparation Time:10 minutes
Cooking time: 40 minutes
Servings: 4
Ingredients:
1 tbsp. miso - 1 tbsp. mirin
1 tbsp. extra virgin Olive oil
skinless cod fillet
red onion, sliced
2 tbsp. celery, sliced
1 clove garlic, finely chopped
1 bird's eye chilli, finely chopped
1tsp fresh ginger, finely chopped
1 cup green beans
¾ cup Kale, roughly chopped
2 tbsp. buckwheat
1tsp ground Turmeric
1tsp sesame seeds
1 tbsp. Parsley, roughly chopped
1 tbsp. tamari or soy sauce
Directions:
Heat the oven to 220ºC/200ºC fan/gas mark 7.
Mix the miso, mirin and 1tsp oil, rub into the cod and Marinate for 30 minutes. Transfer on to a baking tray and cook for 10 minutes.
Meanwhile, heat a large frying pan with the remaining oil. Add the onion and stir-fry for a few minutes, then add the celery, garlic, chilli, ginger, green beans and Kale. Fry until the Kale is tender and cooked through, adding a little water to soften the Kale if needed.
Cook the buckwheat according to pack instructions with the Turmeric. Add the sesame seeds, Parsley and tamari or soy sauce to the stir-fry and serve with the
Nutrition:
Calories: 300g Carbs: 16g Fat: 13g Protein: 30g

Day 6
2 x Sirtfood green juices
2 x Sirtfood meals

150.   Sirt Super Salad

Preparation Time: 5 minutes
Servings: 4
Ingredients:

1 tbsp. rocket
1 tbsp. chicory leaves
1 tbsp. smoked salmon slices
1 tbsp. avocado, peeled, stoned and sliced
2 tbsp. celery, sliced
1 tbsp. red onion, sliced
2 tbsp. walnuts, chopped
1 tbsp. capers
1 large Medjool date, pitted and chopped
1 tbsp. extra virgin Olive oil
Juice 1/2 lemon
1 tbsp. Parsley, chopped
1 tbsp. lovage or celery leaves, chopped

Directions:
Mix all the Ingredients together and serve.

Nutrition:
Calories: 340g
Carbs: 0
Fat: 0
Protein: 30g

151. Chargrilled Beef

Preparation Time: 10 minutes
Cooking time: 45 minutes
Servings: 2
Ingredients:

1 cup potatoes, peeled and diced into 2cm cubes
1 cup extra virgin Olive oil
1 tbsp. Parsley, finely chopped
4 tbsp. red onion, sliced into rings
4 tbsp. Kale, chopped
1 clove garlic, finely chopped
1 cup 3.5cm-thick beef fillet
Steak or 2cm-thick sirloin steak
2 tbsp. red wine
1 cup beef stock
1tsp tomato purée
1tsp cornflour, dissolved in 1tbsp water
Directions:
Heat the oven to 220ºC/200ºC fan/gas mark 7.

Place the potatoes in a saucepan of boiling water, bring to the boil and cook for 4-5 minutes, then Drain. Place in a roasting tin with 1tsp oil and cook for 35-45 minutes, turning every 10 minutes. Remove from the oven, Sprinkle with the chopped Parsley and mix well.

Fry the onion in 1tsp oil over a medium heat until soft and caramelised. Keep warm.
Nutrition:
Calories: 250g
Carbs: 0
Fat: 15g
Protein: 26g

CHAPTER 18:

Sirtfood Chocolate Recipes

152. Delicious Low Carb Brownies with Almond Flour

Preparation Time: 10 minutes
Cooking time: 25 minutes
Servings: 12
Ingredients
50 ml of butter from pasture milk - 50ml Low Carb Schokodrops
3 organic eggs - Pinch of salt - 4 tsp of pure cocoa powder
5 cups almond flour - 4 cups of xylitol
Teaspoon tartar baking powder
A little butter for the baking pan
Directions:
Preheat the oven temperature to 175 ° C top and bottom heat and grease a 20cmx20cm brownie (or a similarly sized casserole dish) with butter.
Melt the butter, and the chocolate drops together inside a water bath.
Separate the eggs.
Beat the egg whites with a little salt.
Using the mixer, stir the cocoa powder under the butter-chocolate mixture. Then add the egg yolk and stir.
Mix almond flour, xylitol, and baking powder and gradually stir into the chocolate mixture. This will be a crumbly mass at first.
Stir in the egg whites and add the batter to the buttered dish and smooth. It works best with wet fingers.
Bake the brownies inside a preheated oven for about 20 - 25 minutes. After baking time, use a wooden stick to test whether the dough is cooked.
Take the brownies from the oven, and then let it cool in the mold. When they are cool, you can take them out of shape.
Tip: Cut into 12-15 pieces and garnish as desired.
Nutrition:
Calories: 215g Carbs: 9 Fat: 18g Protein: 6g

153.   Low Carb Brownie Cheesecake Bites

Preparation Time: 20 minutes
Cooking time: 30 minutes
Servings: 24
Ingredients
For the Bites
Sweet sin chocolate brownies mixture
Soft pasture butter
2 organic eggs
1 cup of water
4 tbsp. water
High-quality ground gelatine
2 cups cream cheese, double cream stage
1 tsp ground vanilla
Birch sugar (xylitol)
Sour cream
1 cup of whipped cream
4 tbsp. of lemon juice
5 tbsp. water
1 cup raspberries
Directions:
Preheat the oven to 150 ° C.
Beat the butter inside a mixing bowl until creamy. Then add the eggs and the water and stir.
Finally, add the baking mixture slowly into the cream and stir until smooth dough is formed.
Layout a spring form pan (diameter 24 cm) with parchment paper or grease with a little butter. Add the dough.
Bake at 150 ° C for 30 minutes. Fresh from the oven, the Sweet Sin Brownie is still incredibly soft, but when cooled, it becomes more stable.
Allow the brownie ground to cool completely.
When the brownie bottom is cold, the cheesecake topping is prepared.
Soak the gelatine in 4 tablespoons of cold water for 10 minutes.
Stir cream cheese with xylitol and vanilla in a creamy bowl. Gradually stir in the sour cream.
Beat the whipped cream inside a separate bowl until stiff.
Heat the lemon juice and 5 tablespoons of water and dissolve the gelatine.

Add two spoons of the cream cheese mixture to the gelatine and stir. Add it to the rest of the cream cheese mixture and stir well.

Stir in the whipped cream quickly and place the mixture on the brownie ground.

for a good 4 hours - better, but overnight - in the fridge.

To release from the mold, let it get a little warm. Cut the cheesecake bites into small pieces and top up with fresh berries as you serve them.

TIP: If you want to cut out the cheesecake bites in the heart shape, they should be slightly frozen beforehand. Otherwise, they will go out of the cookie cutters very badly.

Nutrition:
Calories: 381g
Carbs: 6.7g
Fat: 33g
Protein: 8.68g

154. Protein Chocolate Fudge

Preparation Time:10 minutes
Cooking time: 0 minutes
Servings: 12 balls
Ingredients
5 tsp. cashews
Dates Medjool
Soft plums
2-3 tsp Nutri-Plus Shape & Shake protein powder chocolate
1 tsp. Coconut flower syrup
1 pinch salt
1 knifepoint vanilla
40 g chopped almonds
Directions:
First, add the cashews, the dates (pitted), the plums (pitted), the coconut blossom syrup, the Nutri-Plus protein powder, vanilla with a pinch of salt in a powerful blender.
Mix all ingredients until a homogeneous mixture is obtained.
If your mixer gets too hot, take a break for a while.
Take 1 tablespoon of dough and roll out small balls.
Roll the balls in the almonds (or in cocoa, grated coconut, hazelnuts)
Put the balls inside the fridge for at least 30 minutes to make them firm.
Do not eat all at once!
Nutrition:
Calories: 69.9g
Carbs: 13g
Fat: 1.8g
Protein: 0.4g

155.   Oatmeal Breakfast Pizza

Preparation Time: 10 minutes
Cooking time: 10 minutes
Servings: 1
Ingredients
2 tbsp. oatmeal
15 Nutri-Plus protein powders chocolate
1/2 tsp cinnamon
1 cup Soy yogurt, unsweetened
Something fresh fruit of your choice
Ripe banana
Directions:
Peel a banana and crush it to a pulp with a fork.
Now add the oatmeal, the protein powder, and some cinnamon.
Preheat the oven to 150 ° C and spread the dough in a circle on a baking sheet lined with baking paper.
Leave the dough in the oven for about 10-12 minutes and then cool down a bit so that you can easily remove it from the baking paper.
In the meantime, you can cut your favorite fruit smell.
Distribute the soya yogurt on the oatmeal pizza and top it with the fruit and other toppings of your choice.
Nutrition:
Calories: 260g
Carbs: 29g
Fat: 12g
Protein: 12g

156.   Cookies and Chocolate Tart

Preparation Time: 10 minutes
Cooking time: 1hour
Servings: 2
Ingredients:
Chocolate,
Butter cookies,
And a little milk.
Directions:
We must melt the chocolate and put the cookies in a little bit of milk, before setting the cake floor by floor, alternating a layer of biscuit and chocolate.
Tip: Let it cool before serving
Nutrition:
Calories: 329g
Carbs: 39.5g
Fat: 17.33g
Protein: 5.65g

157.   Easy and Cheap Quick Cookies

Preparation Time: 10 minutes
Cooking time: 25 minutes
Servings: 3
Ingredients
2 cups flour rising
Three eggs
1 1/2 cup sugar
1 cup of butter
One milk splash to knead
Two chocolate bars (I use the eagle bars and cut them)
Directions:
Preheat the oven and prepare a plate in butter and then pass it through the flour. Mix the flour with the sugar
Add to the flour and sugar, the eggs along with the butter, and start mixing.
Incorporate a splash of milk to be able to shape the dough.
Use all the flour needed to knead
Cut the chocolate and incorporate it into the dough. Then
Once ready, cut into small pieces and crush to shape the cookie. Make it as fine as possible because it elevates.
Send it to the oven 200 degrees, only about 5 minutes.
Tip: As with the cake, check with a knife to know if it comes out dry. All these came out; it has made them big socks to take less
Nutrition:
Calories: 181.4g
Carbs: 35.8g
Fat: 62g
Protein: 20.8g

158.   Keto Cookies with Chocolate and Ginger

Preparation Time: 10 minutes
Cooking time: 30 minutes
Servings: 24
Ingredients:
1 cup unsalted butter or
1 cup coconut oil, room warm
1 cup finely powdered erythritol or 120 ml Yacón syrup
1 tsp liquid stevia extract
2 big eggs, whisked
1 cup unsweetened cocoa powder
1 tbsp. cinnamon
2 teaspoons ginger powder
¼ teaspoon fine sea salt
2 teaspoons of vanilla extract
½ teaspoon almond extract

Directions:
Preheat the oven to 175 ° C. Provide two baking trays (do not grease).
Place the butter or coconut oil in a mixing bowl and stir frothy, either with a hand mixer or in the food processor. Add erythritol or yacón syrup and stevia extract and stir thoroughly.
Stir in the eggs, add in the cocoa powder, cinnamon, ginger powder, salt, vanilla, and almond extract and stir the dough again thoroughly.
Form the dough into 5 cm balls and place them on the plates at about 2.5 cm. (The dough diverges when baking it.)
Bake cookies for about 12 minutes till they are cooked through. Let cool on the plate.
Place the cookies in an airtight container for storage. In the refrigerator, they last up to a week in the freezer for up to a month.

Nutrition:
Calories: 157
Carbs: 4.3g
Fat: 0
Protein:5.0g

CHAPTER 19:

Top 14 Sirtfood Recipes

Kickstart your way to a positive lifestyle with this sirtfood diet recipe. The recipes are intended to serve as an example for you so you can be able to create your recipe. This is not a cookbook. These recipes are packed with flavors and foods rich in nutrients that will change the way you eat. Below are the top 21 SIRT recipes.

159.   Baked Salad with Creamy Mint Dressing

Preparation Time: 5 minutes
Cooking time: 20 minutes
Servings: 1
Ingredients
Baked Salmon Salad
4 oz. salmon fillet
2 oz. mixed salad leaves
2 spring onions (finely sliced)
2 radishes (finely sliced)
1 handful of chopped parsley
1 large cucumber (diced into chunks)
Mint Dressing
2 finely chopped mint leaves
1 tsp pure yogurt
Fresh blended black pepper
1 tsp rice vinegar
1 tsp mayonnaise (low-fat)
Salt to taste
Directions:
Preheat oven to 180 C.
Put the salmon fillet on a baking pan and bake for 15 minutes.

While the salmon is in the oven, get a small bowl and pour in the mayonnaise, yogurt, rice vinegar, pepper, mint leaves, salt, and mix. Set aside for a few minutes until you start to perceive the flavors.

On a serving dish, arrange the salmon leaves and spinach, top with parsley, radishes, and red onions nicely.

Toss the cooked salmon on the salad and top with the dressing.

Nutrition:

Calories: 340g

Carbs: 0

Cholesterol: 0

160. Buckwheat Noodles with Chicken, Kale and Miso Dressing

Preparation Time: 5 minutes
Cooking time: 30 minutes
Servings: 3
Ingredients
Noodles
2 handfuls of neatly cut kale leaves - 1 tsp coconut oil
5 oz. whole buckwheat noodles - 1 brown onion (diced)
1 long and thick chili (finely sliced)
2 tbsp Tamari sauce must be gluten-free.
3 sliced shiitake mushrooms
1 medium-size chicken breast (sliced/diced)
2 large garlic cloves (diced) - A few pinches of sea salt to taste
1 Miso Dressing
Tbsp Tamari sauce
1 tbsp lemon juice or lime juice
11/2 tbsp fresh organic miso
1 tbsp extra virgin olive oil
1 tsp sesame oil
Directions:
Boil medium size water in a saucepan. Pour in the kale and allow to boil for a minute, until it is a bit droopy. Remove from the water and keep aside.
Cook the noodles in hot water as directed on the package. Afterward, remove and rinse with cold water and put away.
Heat 1 tsp coconut oil in a frying pan and add in the shiitake mushroom. Allow to brown and add little sea salt and put aside.
Add more coconut oil to the frying pan over slightly high heat. Add the onions and chili pepper and allow to sauté for 2 minutes, 3 minutes max.
Add the chicken afterward into the frying pan and allow it to cook for 5 minutes, with a continuous stir. Pour in the garlic and the Tamari sauce and add a little water. Leave to cook for 2 minutes and keep striving until the chicken is tenderly cooked. Add the kale and buckwheat noodles and stir together. Mix the miso dressing and spread on the noodles when you are about ending the cooking.
Nutrition:
Calories: 454 Carbohydrates: 21g Fat: 28 Protein: 38g

161.   Asian King Prawn Stir Fry with Buckwheat Noodles

Preparation Time: 5 minutes
Cooking time: 15 minutes
Servings: 1
Ingredients
5 oz. shelled prawn, raw king to be precise.
2.5 oz. buckwheat noodles
2 tsp Tamari sauce (gluten free)
2 bird's eye chilies
100ml chicken stock
3 tsp extra virgin olive oil
1 garlic clove (chopped)
1 tsp ginger (chopped)
1.5 oz. kale (chopped)
2.5 oz. green beans
1 red onion (sliced)
1 celery leaf
2 celery leaves (sliced)

Directions:
Cooking noodles in boiling water as instructed on the package. When it's tenderly cooked, drain and keep aside.

Bring a frying pan to heat over medium heat, add the prawns, 1 teaspoon each of the tamari sauce and extra virgin olive oil, and allow cooking for 3 minutes. Remove the prawns from the pan and set aside. Clean the pan with a kitchen wipe.

Add the remaining oil to the frying pan and pour in the garlic, ginger, red onion, chili pepper, kale, green beans, celery and allow to fry over medium heat for about 3 minutes.

Pour in the stock and allow the vegetable to cook thoroughly and taste crunchy.

Add the noodles, prawns, celery leaves to the mixed vegetables and allow them to simmer for a few minutes.

Remove from the heat and serve hot.

Nutrition:
Total Fat: 11.2g Carbohydrate: 1.6g
Trans Fat: 0g Protein: 70g

162.   Coronation Chicken Salad

Preparation Time: 5 minutes
Servings: 1
Ingredients
4 oz. cooked breast chicken, cut into small pieces
1 tsp blended turmeric
2.5 oz. pure yogurt
1 bird's eye chili
1 tsp chopped coriander
¼ lemon juice
6 ½ walnuts (chopped)
½ tsp curry
1 oz. rocket (for serving)
2 medium-size red onions (diced)
1 Medjool date (neatly chopped)
Directions:
Mix the yogurt, spices, coriander, lemon juice in a clean bowl and mix gently.
Add all the other ingredients and mix them.
Serve with rocket.
Nutrition:
Total Fat: 180
Carbohydrate: 8.7g
Fat: 14.3g
Protein: 3.70g

163.   Sirtfood Mushroom Scramble Eggs

Preparation Time: 2 minutes
Cooking time: 10 minutes
Servings: 1
Ingredients
1 oz. kale (chopped)
A large handful of parsley (chopped)
2 eggs
1 tsp curry
A handful of sliced button mushroom
1 tsp extra virgin olive oil
1 tsp turmeric
½ bird's eye chili
Directions:
Mix in a bowl the curry pans turmeric powder. Add a little water and mix till you get a nice and smooth paste.
Bring kale to steam for about 3 minutes.
Pour the olive oil in a frying pan and allow it to heat, and then pour in the bird's eye chili and mushroom and leave to fry for 2 minutes. Allow turning brown, then add the eggs, above paste, and leave to simmer. Add the kale and leave to cook for a few more minutes.
Nutrition:
Total Fat: 182
Carbohydrate: 4g
Fat: 12g
Protein: 12g

164.   Sesame Chicken Salad

Preparation Time: 2 minutes
Cooking time: 10 minutes
Servings: 2
Ingredients
3 oz. baby kale (chopped)
A large handful of parsley (chopped)
1 tbsp sesame seed
½ red onions (sliced)
5 oz. of chicken (cooked and shredded)
1 cucumber, peeled, with no seed and sliced.
2 oz. Pak choi
Dressing
1 tsp sesame oil
1 tsp honey
1 tsp extra virgin olive oil
2 tsp soy sauce
1 lime (juiced)
Directions:
Pour the sesame seed in a frying pan and allow it to fry for like 2 minutes thereabout. Remove from frying pan when it's slightly brown and set aside.
Mix the remaining sesame oil, olive oil, honey, lime juice, and soy sauce in a bowl and set aside. This is the Dressing.
Pour the Pak choi, cucumber, parsley, kale, and red onion in another mixing bowl and mix. Add the dressing mix with this and mix it until it's well combined.
Pour the sesame seed. Serve and add the shredded chicken.
Nutrition:
Total Fat: 330
Carbohydrate: 13g
Fat: 19g
Protein: 30g

165.   Smoked Salmon Omelette

Preparation Time: 2 minutes
Cooking time: 10 minutes
Servings: 1
Ingredients
3.5 oz. smoked salmon (sliced)
0.35 oz. chopped rocket
1 tsp extra virgin olive oil
2 medium size eggs
½ capers
1 tsp parsley.
Directions:
Break the eggs in a bowl and whisk gently.
Pour into the egg capers, parsley, salmon, rocket, and mix well.
Heat the olive oil in a frying pan and allow it to get extremely hot. Then, pour the egg in the hot oil and spread evenly with a spatula
Reduce the heat to low and leave to cook.
Use the spatula to smooth the edges and fold the omelet into two, then serve.
Nutrition:
Total Fat: 202
Carbohydrate: 0g
Fat: 13g
Protein: 19g

166. Salmon Sirt Salad

Preparation Time: 2 minutes
Cooking time: 5 minutes
Servings: 2
Ingredients
1.6 oz. rocket
0.35 oz. chopped parsley
0.35 oz. chopped celery leaves
1 large tbsp Medjool date
0.7 oz. sliced red onion
0.5 oz. chopped walnuts
¼ lemon juice
1 tsp capers
1 tsp extra virgin olive oil
2.8 oz. chopped avocado
3.5 oz. smoked salmon
0.7 oz. sliced celery
Directions:
Arrange all the salad leaves on a large serving plate.
Add the other ingredients in mixing bowl and mix gently.
Serve the mixture on the leaves.
Nutrition:
Total Fat: 202
Carbohydrate: 5g
Fat: 3g
Carbs: 8g

167.   Sirt Muesli

Preparation Time: 5 minutes
Serves: 2
Ingredients
0.7 oz. buckwheat flakes
3.5 oz. Plain Greek yogurt
0.7 oz. Medjool date (finely chopped)
0.35 oz. cocoa nibs
3.5 oz. chopped strawberries
0.5 oz. Coconut flakes
9.35 buckwheat puffs
Directions:
In a large mixing bowl, pour in all the ingredients, leaving out the yogurt ad strawberries until when you are ready to serve it.
Nutrition:
Total Fat: 280
Carbohydrate: 43g
Fat: 6g
Protein: 10g

168.   Sirt Fruit Salad

Preparation Time: 10 minutes
Serves: 1
Ingredients
Half a cup of fresh green tea
10 blueberries
1 orange
10 red grapes, seedless
1 Apple, chopped and cored
1 tsp honey
Directions:
Add the honey into the green tea and stir. Add the orange juice from half of the orange and keep inside the fridge to cool.
Chop the remaining orange in a clean bowl; add all the remaining ingredients and mix.
Bring out the green tea from the fridge and put the mixture on it. Set aside too steep for a while.
Serve when adequately steeped.
Nutrition:
Total Fat: 110
Carbohydrate: 17g
Fat: 0g
Protein: 2g

169. Kale and Black Currant Smoothie

Preparation Time: 5 minutes
Serves: 1
Ingredients
A cup of warm green tea
1 ripe banana
2 tsp honey
6 ice cubes
10 baby kale leaves, without stalk
1.4 oz. blackcurrant
Directions:
Add honey to the green tea and stir.
Add all the ingredients together in a food processor and blend.
Serve cold.
Nutrition:
Total Fat: 972
Carbohydrate: 127g
Fat: 48g
Protein: 25g

170.   Green Tea Smoothie

Preparation Time: 5 minutes
Serves: 1
Ingredients
2 tsp matcha green tea powder
A pack of milk
2 tsp honey
2 ripe bananas
6 ice cubes
½ vanilla bean paste
Directions:
Blend all the ingredients in a food processor and serve.
Nutrition:
Total Fat: 300
Carbohydrate: 50g
Fat: 5g
Protein: 20g

171.   Turmeric Baked Salmon

Preparation Time: 20 minutes
Serves: 2
Ingredients
5 oz. skinned salmon
¼ lemon juice
1 tsp turmeric
1 tsp extra virgin olive oil
Spicy Sauce
0.5 oz. celery
1 garlic clove
1 large chopped red onion
1 tsp curry powder
1 large tomato, diced into 8 pieces
1 tsp extra virgin olive oil
1 tsp parsley, finely chopped
A medium-size canned green bean
1 bird's eye chili
100ml Chicken stock
Small chopped fresh ginger
Directions:
Heat oven at 180 C.
Add olive oil to a frying pan and allow to heat on low heat. Add the onions, celery, garlic, chili, ginger, and fry for 2 minutes. Mix in the curry powder and allow to cook for a few seconds.
Pour in the tomatoes, green beans, and chicken stock and leave to simmer for few more minutes.
Mix the lemon juice, olive oil, and turmeric and apply the mixture on the salmon. Arrange on a baking tray and bake for 10 minutes.
Sprinkle the spicy parsley sauce and serve with the salmon.
Nutrition:
Total Fat: 143
Carbohydrate: 0g
Fat: 6g
Protein: 22g

172.   Buckwheat Pasta Salad

Cooking time: 5 minutes.
Serves: 1
Ingredients
1.75 oz. buckwheat pasta
A handful of rockets
Half sliced avocado
0.7 oz. pine nuts
10 olives
8 cherry tomatoes
1 tsp extra virgin olive oil
Small handful basil leaves
Directions:
Mix all the ingredients in a bowl, leaving out the pine nuts. When thoroughly mixed, sprinkle the pine nuts on top. Then serve.
Nutrition:
Total Fat: 220
Carbohydrate: 46g
Fat: 0g
Protein:8g

CHAPTER 20:

Super Sirtfood Diet Main Recipe

173.   Tuscan Carrot Bean Stew

Preparation Time:10 minutes
Cook time: 40 minutes
Servings: 1
Ingredients
2 tbsp. of buckwheat - 1 cup of roughly chopped parsley
2 tbsp. of kale, roughly chopped - 1 cup of tinned mixed beans
1 tsp of tomato purée - 1 cup of tin chopped Italian tomatoes
2 cups of vegetable stock - 1 tsp of herbs de Provence
(Optional) half bird's eye chili, finely chopped
1 finely chopped garlic clove
2 tbsp. of celery, trimmed and finely chopped
2 tbsp. grams of peeled and chopped carrot
4 tbsp. of finely chopped red onion
1 tbsp. of extra virgin olive oil
Directions:
Gently fry the onion, celery, carrot, chili (if using), garlic, and herbs in hot oil over low–medium heat in a medium saucepan until the onion is soft.
Add the tomato purée, vegetable stock, and tomatoes and bring to a boil. Pour in beans and simmer about 30 minutes.
Add chopped kale and cook for an additional 6 to 10 minutes, until kale is soft, add in chopped parsley.
Cook the buckwheat the way instructed in packet directions, drain. Serve cooked buckwheat noodles with bean stew.
Nutrition:
Total Fat: 109.1 Carbohydrate: 17.8g Fat: 2.4g Protein: 5.3g

174.   Chicken and Turmeric Salad

Preparation Time: 12 minutes
Cook time: 15 minutes
Servings: 1
Ingredients
1 handful of coriander chopped leaves - 1 handful of parsley chopped
1/2 sliced avocado - 2 tbsp of pumpkin seeds
3 large kale leaves (cut off stems) - 2 cups of broccoli florets
Juice of 1/2 lime - 1 tsp of lime zest
9-oz of diced up chicken breast
1/2 diced onion - 1 tsp of turmeric powder
1 tbsp of coconut oil - 1 large minced garlic clove
For the Dressing
½ tsp of sea salt and pepper
½ tsp of wholegrain or Dijon mustard
1 tsp of raw honey
3 tbsp of extra-virgin olive oil
1 small grated garlic clove, or finely diced
3 tbsp of lime juice
Directions:
Heat the coconut oil over medium heat in a frying pan. Sauté onion in hot oil for 4 minutes until soft and fragrant. Add in garlic and chicken pieces to the frying pan, cook stirring for about 2 to 3 minutes, and breaking apart. Add lime zest and juice, salt, turmeric, and pepper; allow cooking for an extra 3 to 4 minutes. Transfer to a bowl and set aside.
Cook the broccoli florets in boiling water in a small saucepan for 2-3 minutes, rinse with cold water.
Pour the pumpkin seeds into the same frying pan earlier used in cooking the chicken. Toast for a few minutes over medium heat, stirring continuously, so it does not burn.
Combine the dressing ingredients in a bowl. Place kale into a large salad bowl and spread the dressing over kale in the bowl, tossing until coated. Add in chicken, broccoli florets, herbs, pumpkin seeds, avocado slices, parsley, and coriander and toss to coat well.
Nutrition:
Total Fat: 66 Carbohydrate: 2g Fat: 2g Protein: 6g

175. Baked Cod Marinated in Miso with Greens

Preparation Time: 50 minutes
Cook time: 25 minutes
Servings: 1
Ingredients
1 tsp of ground turmeric
1/4 cup of buckwheat (40g)
1 tbsp of soy sauce
2 tbsp of roughly chopped parsley, (5g)
1 tsp of sesame seeds
3/4 cup of roughly chopped kale, (50g)
3/8 cup of green beans (60g)
1 tsp of finely chopped fresh ginger
1 finely chopped Thai chili
2 finely chopped garlic cloves
3/8 cup of sliced celery, (40g)
1/8 cup of sliced red onion, (20g)
1 x 7-oz of the skinless cod fillet (200g)
1 tbsp of extra virgin olive oil
1 tbsp of mirin
(20g) 3 1/2 tsp of miso

Directions:
Mix 1 tsp of olive oil, miso, and mirin. Rub the cod all over with the mixture and let it marinate for a half-hour.

Preheat the oven to 425 degrees F. Once you are done marinating, place the cod in the oven and bake for 10 minutes.

While the cod is cooking, pour the remaining olive oil in a large frying pan and heat over medium heat. Stir-fry the onion in the hot oil for a few minutes; add the ginger, celery, kale, garlic, green beans, and chili. Cook stirring frequently and tossing until the kale is cooked through and tender. Add a few drops of water to the pan if needed.

Cook the buckwheat along with turmeric the way instructed in package instruction.

Add the soy sauce, parsley, and sesame seeds to the stir-fry. Serve fish with the stir-fry and buckwheat.

Nutrition:
Total Fat: 222 Carbohydrate: 21.7g Fat: .9g Protein: 25.4g

176. Chicken Breast with Chili Salsa and Red Onions

Preparation Time: 10 minutes
Cook time: 20 minutes
Servings: 1
Ingredients
4 tbsp. of buckwheat - 1 tsp of chopped fresh ginger
1 tbsp. of sliced red onion - 4 tbsp. of chopped kale
1 tbsp. of extra virgin olive oil - ¼ lemon juice
2 tsp of ground turmeric - 1 cup of boneless, skinless chicken breast
For the salsa
¼ lemons Juice
1 tbsp. finely chopped parsley - 1 tbsp. of capers, finely chopped
1 finely chopped bird's eye chili - 1 cup of tomato
Directions:
How to Make the Salsa:
Finely chop the tomato, trying to keep as much of the juice as you can.
Mix the chopped tomato with the parsley, lemon juice, capers, and chili.
Preheat the oven to 425 F. In a bowl, mix a little olive oil, 1 tsp. Turmeric and lemon juice. Place the chicken breast and marinate for 5–10 minutes.
Meanwhile, heat an oven-resistance frying pan over medium-high heat until hot, place the chicken and cook until pale golden, about 1 to 1 1/2 minutes on each side.
Place the frying pan in the oven and bake until cooked through, for 8–10 minutes. Place pan on a baking tray if you did not use a heat-proof pan. Once cooked, remove chicken from the oven, cover with foil, and let sit for five minutes before carving.
While the chicken is cooking, add the kale to a steamer and cook for 5 minutes.
Add a little oil to a frying pan and cook the ginger and red onions until soft but not colored. Add in the cooked kale to the frying pan and cook for an additional 1 minute.
Cook the buckwheat along with the remaining turmeric the way instructed in package instruction. (Takes about 5-8 minutes) Serve the chicken alongside the buckwheat, vegetables, and salsa.
Nutrition:
Total Fat: 142 Carbohydrate: 3g Fat: 3g Protein: 33g

177.   Mushrooms with Buckwheat Kasha and Olives

Preparation Time: 5 minutes
Cook time: 20 minutes
Servings: 4
Ingredients
1/4 cup of chopped parsley
1/2 cup of black olives sliced
¾ cup of baby Bella mushrooms
1 tbsp of olive oil
1 tbsp of almond butter
1 cup of buckwheat groats toasted
2 teaspoon salt
2 tbsp of soy sauce
Directions:
Add 2 cups of water, buckwheat, butter, and salt in a pot. Bring mixture to a boil, turn the heat down and simmer for 20 minutes with the lid on.
Add the olive oil to a pan over medium-high heat. Add in the mushrooms and fry about 10-15 minutes or until lightly browned.
Combine the mushrooms/buckwheat mix, olives, soy sauce, and parsley Mix In a large bowl.
Nutrition:
Total Fat: 142
Carbohydrate: 3g
Fat: 3g
Protein: 33g

178.   Asian Prawn Tofu

Preparation Time: 10 minutes
Cook time: 15 minutes
Servings: 5
Ingredients
1 tbsp. of good-quality miso paste
1 tbsp. of sushi ginger, chopped
2 tbsp. of cooked water chestnuts, drained
2 tbsp. of rice noodles
chopped firm tofu
1 cup of raw tiger prawns
2 tbsp. of bean sprouts
2 tbsp. of broccoli, cut into small florets
1/2 carrot, cut into matchsticks
4 cups of fresh chicken stock, or made with 1 cube
Juice of 1/2 lime
A small handful of coriander stalks finely chopped (.35oz.)
A small handful of parsley stalks finely chopped (.35oz.)
1 crushed star anise, or 1/4 tsp of ground anise
1 tsp of tomato purée
Directions:
In a large pan, add the chicken stock, star anise, tomato purée, parsley stalks, lime juice, and coriander stalks and bring mixture to a simmer, about 10 minutes.
Cook the rice noodles according to packet instructions, drain.
Add cooked noodles, broccoli, tofu, carrot, prawns, and water chestnuts and gently simmer until the vegetables and prawns are cooked. Turn heat off and stir in the miso paste and sushi ginger. Serve with a sprinkle of coriander and parsley.
Nutrition:
Total Fat: 170
Carbohydrate: 11g
Fat: 8.5g
Protein: 14.1g

179.   Potatoes and Grilled Beef

Preparation Time:20 minutes
Cook time: 70 minutes
Servings: 1
Ingredients
1 cup grams of potatoes, peeled and diced into 2cm cubes
1 tbsp. of extra virgin olive oil - 1 tbsp. of parsley, finely chopped
4 tbsp. of red onion, sliced into rings - 4 tbsp. of kale, chopped
1 clove garlic, finely chopped - 1 cup of beef fillet, 3.5cm-thick
Steak or 2 cm-thick sirloin steak - 2 tbsp. red wine
1 cup of beef stock - 1 tsp of tomato purée
1 tsp of corn flour, disso
Directions:
Preheat the oven to 220ºC.
Bring water to a boil in a saucepan and cook the potatoes for about 4-5 minutes, then drain.
Add 1 teaspoon of olive oil in the roasting tin and cook the potatoes in the oven about 35 to 45 minutes, turning every 10 minutes. Withdraw the potatoes from the oven, sprinkle well with chopped parsley, and mix well.
Fry the onion in 1 teaspoon of olive in a frying pan over medium heat until tender and caramelized. Keep warm.
Steam the kale for 2-3 minutes in boiling water in a medium saucepan until slightly wilted, then drain. Gently sauté the garlic in half teaspoon of olive oil until soft, about 1 minute. Add in kale and cook until soft, 1-2 minutes. Keep warm.
Heat an oven-safe pan over medium heat until hot. Coat the meat in half teaspoon of olive oil and fry to your desired likeness. Set aside to rest.
Pour red wine into the hot frying pan and deglaze any brown bit from the pan. Cook until liquid is reduced by half and syrupy with a concentrated flavor.
Add tomato purée and beef stock into the pan, bring mixture to the boil.
Slowly add the corn flour paste into the pan to thicken the sauce until you have your desired consistency. Stir in any juice from the rested steak and serve with potatoes, kale, onion rings, and red wine sauce
Nutrition:
Total Fat: 220 Carbohydrate: 30g Fat: 2g Protein: 21g

180.   Butternut, Lamb Tagine

Preparation Time: 15 minutes
Cook time: 1 hour 15 minutes
Servings: 4
Ingredients
2 tbsp. of freshly chopped coriander, plus more for garnish
1 cup of tin chickpeas, drained
4 cups of butternut squash, chopped into 1 cm cubes
1 cup of chopped tomatoes tin, plus 1/2 of the liquid from a can
1 cup of Medjool dates, pitted and chopped
½ tsp of salt - 3 ½ cup of lamb neck fillet, cut into 2cm pieces
2 tsp of ground turmeric - 1 cinnamon stick - 2 tsp of cumin seeds
1 tsp of chili flakes - 3 grated garlic cloves, or crushed
2 cm ginger, grated - 1 sliced red onion - 2 tbsp. of olive oil
Directions:
Heat-up the oven to 285 F.
In a cast-iron skillet or a large oven-safe saucepan with lid, heat about 2 tbsp. of olive oil. Gently cook the onion in hot oil for about 5 minutes, with the lid on until onions are tender but not brown.
Add the ginger and grated garlic, cumin, turmeric, cinnamon, and chili. Stir together and cook without the lid for 1 extra minute. You can add a little bit of water to help with the cooking if you feel it's too dry.
Add in the lamb pieces, stirring thoroughly so the meat coat in the spices. Add the chopped dates, salt, and tomatoes with half of the liquid from can (100-200ml).
Bring to a boil, place the lid, then transfer to the preheated oven and cook for 75 minutes.
Remove from oven 30 minutes before the final cooking time and add in the drained chickpeas and chopped squash. Stir until everything is well mixed, cover and place back in the oven; cook for the last 30 minutes.
Once it's cooked, withdraw and stir in the coriander; best served with flatbreads, buckwheat, basmati rice, or couscous.
Nutrition:
Total Fat: 479
Carbohydrate: 9g
Fat: 28g
Protein: 45g

CHAPTER 21:

Vegan Recipes

181.   Veggie Chili and Baked Potato

Preparation Time: 10 minutes
Serves 1
Ingredients
Kidney beans - ½ cup
Black beans - ½ cup
Crushed chunky tomatoes - 1 cup
Corn - 1/4 cup
Zucchini - ½ cup (chopped)
Ground cumin - 1 teaspoon
Onion - 1/4 cup (diced)
Chili powder - 1 teaspoon
Nonfat plain Greek yogurt - ¼ cup
Baked potato - 1 medium-size
Heat your oven to 350 degrees F.
Use a fork or a knife to poke holes
Directions:
On the top of the potato, and then place it in the oven to bake for about 30 to 40 minutes, until soft.
Place a pot over medium heat. Add the onions, zucchini, spices, tomatoes, corn, and beans. Stir—Cook for about 15 minutes.
Place the baked potato and chili on a plate and top with Greek yogurt.
Nutrition:
Total Fat: 380
Carbohydrate: 61g
Fat: 10g
Protein: 17g

182.   Parsley Smoothie

Preparation Time: 2 minutes
Serves 2
Ingredients
Flat-leaf parsley - 1 cup
Juice of two lemons
Apple – 1 (core removed)
Avocado – 1
Chopped kale - 1 cup
Peeled fresh ginger – 1 knob
Honey or maple syrup- 1 tablespoon
Iced water - 2 cups
Directions:
Add all the ingredients except the avocado into your blender. Blend on high until smooth, then add the avocado, then set your blender to slow speed and blend until creamy. Add a little more iced water if the smoothie is too thick.
Nutrition:
Total Fat: 239
Carbohydrate: 61g
Fat: 0g
Protein: 3g

183.   Matcha Overnight Oats

Preparation Time: 10 minutes
Cooking time: 10 minutes
Servings: 2
Ingredients
For the Oats
Chia seeds - 2 teaspoon
Rolled oats – 3 oz.
Matcha powder - 1 teaspoon
Honey or maple syrup - 1 teaspoon
Almond milk – 1 ½ cups
Ground cinnamon - 2 pinches
For the Topping
Apple – 1 (peeled, cored and chopped)
A handful of mixed nuts
Pumpkin seeds – 1 teaspoon
Directions:
Get your oats ready a night before. Place the chia seeds and the oats in a container or bowl.
In a different jug or bowl, add the matcha powder and one tablespoon of almond milk and whisk with a hand-held mixer until you get a smooth paste, then add the rest of the milk and mix thoroughly.
Pour the milk mixture over the oats, add the honey and cinnamon, and then stir well. Cover the bowl with a lid and place in the fridge overnight.
When you want to eat, transfer the oats to two serving bowls, then top with the nuts, pumpkin seeds, and chopped apple.
Nutrition:
Total Fat: 320
Carbohydrate: 38g
Fat: 11g
Protein: 21g

184. Homemade Kale Chips

Preparation Time: 10 minutes
Cook time: 14 minutes
Serves: 2 to 4
Ingredients
Kale – 140g (stalks taken off, washed and dried)
Chili flakes - ½ teaspoon
Dried garlic granules - 1 teaspoon
Salt - ½ teaspoon
Nutritional yeast flakes - 1 tablespoon
Extra virgin olive oil - 1 tablespoon
Directions:
Heat your oven to 300 degrees F.
Wash the kale clean and dry the leaves very well. Remove the woody stalks and break into bite-size pieces.
Place the kale into a bowl; sprinkle the remaining ingredients plus the olive oil. Use your fingers to massage the ingredients into the kale until well coated.
Place the coated kale into two baking trays while ensuring that the leaves do not overlap.
Cook for approx. Seven minutes, then rotate the tray and cook for another 7 minutes.
Allow to cool a little before you serve.
Nutrition:
Total Fat: 20
Carbohydrate: 6g
Fat: 2g
Protein: 1g

185. Buckwheat Pita Bread Sirtfood

Preparation Time: 10 minutes
Cooking time: 15 minutes
Servings: 6
Ingredients
Packet dried yeast - 1 x 1 tbsp.
Lukewarm water
Extra virgin olive oil – 3 tbsp.
Buckwheat flour – 2 cups
Sea salt - 1 teaspoon
Polenta for dusting
Directions:
Add the yeast in the lukewarm water, mix and set aside for about 10 to 15 minutes to activate.
Mix the buckwheat flour, olive oil, salt, and yeast mixture. Work slowly to make dough. Cover and place in a warm spot for approx. One hour – this is to get the dough to rise.
Divide the dough into six parts—sharpen one of the pieces into a flat disc and place between two sheets of a baking paper. Gently roll out the dough into a round pita shape that is approximately ¼-inch thick.
Use a fork to pierce the dough a few times, and then dust lightly with polenta.
Heat your cast iron pan and brush the pan with olive oil. Cook the pita for about 5 minutes on one side until puffy, and then turn to the other side and repeat.
Fill the pita with your preferred veggies, then serve immediately.
Nutrition:
Total Fat: 100
Carbohydrate: 20g
Fat: 0g
Protein: 3g

186.   Coronation Tofu Salad

Preparation Time:10 minutes
Servings: 2
Ingredients
Cooked tofu – 100g (cut into bite-sized pieces)
Natural yogurt – ½ cup
Arugula – 1.5 oz., to serve
Ground turmeric - 1 teaspoon
Juice of 1/4 of a lemon
Medjool date – 1 (finely chopped)
Coriander - 1 teaspoon (chopped)
Mild curry powder - ½ teaspoon
Walnut halves – 6 (finely chopped)
Bird's eye chili – 1
Red onion – 1/3 cup (diced)
Directions:
Add the spices, coriander, lemon juice, and yogurt in a bowl. Mix, then add the remaining ingredients and serve on a bed of arugula.
Nutrition:
Total Fat: 326
Carbohydrate: 28.7g
Fat: 13g
Protein: 28.4g

CHAPTER 22:

Vegetarian Recipes

187.   Buckwheat Pasta Salad

Preparation Time: 5 minutes
Servings: 2
Ingredients
A large handful of rockets (arugula)
Cooked buckwheat pasta - ¾ cup
Avocado - ½ (diced)
Small handful of basil leaves
Extra virgin olive oil - 1 tablespoon
Cherry tomatoes – 8 (halved)
Olives - 10
Pine nuts – 1/3 cup
Directions:
Add all the ingredients except the pine nuts into a bowl and mix. Arrange the mixture in a bowl or plate, and then scatter the pine nuts on top.
Nutrition:
Total Fat: 220
Carbohydrate: 46g
Fat: 0g
Protein: 8g

188.　　Greek Salad Skewers

Preparation Time: 10 minutes
Servings: 2
Ingredients
Wooden skewers – 2 (soak in water for thirty minutes before you use)
Cherry tomatoes - 8
Cucumber – 3.5-oz (cut into four slices and halved)
Large black olives - 8
Yellow pepper - 1 (cut into eight squares)
Feta - 3.5-oz (cut into eight cubes)
Red onion - ½ (cut in half and separated into eight pieces)
For the Dressing
Extra virgin olive oil - 1 tablespoon
Balsamic vinegar - 1 teaspoon
Juice of half a lemon
Garlic - ½ clove (peeled and crushed)
Few leaves oregano, finely chopped
Few leaves basil, finely chopped
Freshly ground pepper and salt, to season
Directions:
Thread each of the skewers with the salad ingredients in the following order: olive, yellow pepper, tomatoes, red onion, cucumber, feta, olive, tomato, yellow pepper, cucumber, red onion, and feta.
Mix all the dressing ingredients in a small bowl, and then pour over the skewers.
Nutrition:
Total Fat: 236
Carbohydrate: 14g
Fat: 21g
Protein: 7g

189.   Edamame, Kale and Tofu Curry

Preparation Time:10 minutes
Cooking time: 45minutes
Servings: 4
Ingredients
Firm tofu – 1 cup (chopped into cubes)
Frozen soya edamame beans - ¾ cup
Tomatoes - 2 (roughly chopped)
Kale leaves – 1 cup (stalks removed and torn)
Rapeseed oil - 1 tablespoon
Large onion - 1 (chopped)
Ground turmeric - ½ teaspoon
Garlic - 4 cloves (peeled and grated)
Fresh ginger - 1 large thumb (peeled and grated)
Red chili – 1 (deseeded and thinly sliced)
Paprika - 1 teaspoon
Cayenne pepper - 1/4 teaspoon
Ground cumin - ½ teaspoon
Salt - 1 teaspoon
Dried red lentils – 1 cup
Juice of 1 lime
Boiling water - 1 liter
Directions:
Add the oil into a heavy-bottomed pan, placed over low-medium heat. Add the onions and cook for approx. 5 minutes, then add the chili, ginger, and garlic. Cook for another 2 minutes. Add the salt, cumin, paprika, cayenne, and turmeric. Stir through before you add the red lentils and stir again.

Add the boiling water to the pan and allow it to simmer for ten minutes, then reduce the heat and cook for another 30 minutes until the curry gets a thick porridge-like consistency.

Add the tomatoes, tofu, and beans. Cook for another 5 minutes. Add the kale leaves and the lime juice. Cook until the kale turns tender. Serve.
Nutrition:
Total Fat: 119
Carbohydrate: 7g
Fat: 6g
Protein: 8g

190.   Sesame Tofu Salad

Preparation Time: 12 minutes
Servings: 2
Ingredients
Cooked tofu – 0.625g (shredded)
Cucumber – 1 (peel, halve lengthways, deseed with a teaspoon and slice)
Sesame seeds - 1 tablespoon
Baby kale - 0.4375 g (roughly chopped)
Red onion – ½ (shredded finely)
Pak choi – ½ cup (shredded finely)
Large handful (20g) parsley, chopped
For the Dressing
Soy sauce - 2 teaspoon
Sesame oil - 1 teaspoon
Extra virgin olive oil - 1 tablespoon
Juice of 1 lime
Honey or maple syrup- 1 teaspoon
Directions:
Toast the sesame seeds in a dry frypan for approx. Two minutes until fragrant and lightly browned. Transfer the seeds to a plate to cool.
Mix the lime juice, soy sauce, honey, sesame oil, and olive oil in a small bowl to get your dressing.
Place the Pak choi, parsley, red onion, kale, and cucumber in a large bowl. Mix. Add to the bowl of the dressing and mix again.
Share the salad into two plates, and then add the shredded tofu on top. Sprinkle over the sesame seeds before you serve.
Nutrition:
Total Fat: 200
Carbohydrate: 8g
Fat: 12g
Protein: 20g

191.   Sirtfood Mushroom and Scramble Eggs

Preparation Time: 10 minutes
Cooking time: 10 minutes
Servings: 1
Ingredients
Kale – 1 tbsp. (roughly chopped)
Eggs - 2
Mild curry powder - 1 teaspoon
Ground turmeric - 1 teaspoon
Extra virgin olive oil - 1 teaspoon
Bird's eye chili - ½ (thinly sliced)
Parsley – 1 tbsp. (finely chopped)
Directions:
Add a little water into a bowl; add the curry powder, and turmeric. Mix until you have a light paste.
Steam the kale for about 3 minutes.
Place a frypan over medium heat, add the oil to heat, and then add the mushrooms and chili, fry for about 3 minutes until they start to brown and soften.
Enjoy
Nutrition:
Total Fat: 186.9
Carbohydrate: 2.6g
Fat: 14.3g
Protein: 12.0g

192.   Aromatic Tofu with Salsa, Red Onion and Kale

Cooking time: 2 hours
Servings: 2
Ingredients
Firm tofu – 0.5g - Juice of ¼ lemon
Ground turmeric - 2 teaspoon
Kale - ¾ cup (chopped) - Extra virgin olive oil - 1 tablespoon
Red onion - 1/8 cup (sliced)
Buckwheat - 1/3 cup
Chopped fresh ginger - 1 teaspoon
For the Salsa
Thai chili – 1 (finely chopped)
Medium tomato – 1
Capers - 1 tablespoon (finely chopped)
Juice of ¼ lemon
Parsley - 2 tablespoons (finely chopped)
Directions:
To prepare the salsa, remove the eyes of the tomato and chop it very finely, preserving as much of the liquid as possible. Add the chopped tomato, lemon juice, parsley, capers, and chili into a bowl and mix.
Heat the oven to 220ºC or 425 degrees F. Mix one teaspoon of turmeric, a little oil and lemon juice in a bowl, and then marinate the tofu with the mixture. Leave for about five to ten minutes.
Place an ovenproof frying pan on medium heat until hot, then add the marinated tofu and cook for about one minute on each side until it turns pale golden before you transfer the tofu to the oven for about 5 mins or until well cooked. If you do not have an ovenproof pan, cook the tofu in your regular pan and then place it on a baking tray and keep in the oven until well cooked. Remove from the oven, wrap with a foil, and keep aside to rest for five minutes before you serve.
While waiting, steam the kale for 5 minutes. Fry the ginger and red onions in a little oil, until the onion turns soft but not colored, then add the cooked kale and cook for an extra one minute.
Cook the buckwheat following the instructions on the packet, add the remaining teaspoon of turmeric. Serve alongside the salsa, veggies, and tofu.
Nutrition:
Total Fat: 490 Carbohydrate: 63g Fat: 18g Protein:19g

CHAPTER 23:

Healthy Sirtfood Diet Recipes

193.   Apple Green Ceviche

Preparation Time: 10 minutes
Cooking time: 20 minutes
Servings:2
Ingredients
1/4 cup of lemon juice - 1/3 cup of orange juice
2 tablespoons of olive oil - 1/4 bunch of coriander
2 pieces of green apple without peel cut into medium cubes
1 piece of finely chopped serrano chili
1 cup of jicama cut into medium cubes
1 piece of avocado cut into cubes
1 cup cucumber cut into cubes
1/4 bunch of finely chopped basil leaf
1/4 cup of finely chopped cilantro
1 pinch of salt
1 piece of sliced radish
1 piece of serrano chili cut into slices
1/4 piece of purple onion
Directions:
Add lemon juice, orange juice, olive oil, and cilantro to the blender. Blend perfectly well. Reservation.
Add to a bowl the apple, serrano pepper, jicama, avocado, cucumber, basil, cilantro, mix with the Directions: of the blender and season perfectly well.
Serve the ceviche in a deep dish and decorate with the radish the Chile serrano and the purple onion. Enjoy
Nutrition:
Total Fat: 885 Carbohydrate: 83.7g Fat: 14.3g Protein: 117g

194.   Soup 'green

Preparation Time:30 minutes
Servings: 1
Ingredients:
Water in sufficient quantity to achieve the desired texture
1 green apple with skin
1 slice of fresh peeled ginger
Half lemon or 1 lime without skin, the white part without seeds
Half cucumber with skin
Half bowl of leaves with fresh spinach
1 bunch of basil or fresh cilantro
1 branch of wireless celery, including tender green
Leaves
Directions:
Wash and chop all the ingredients. Insert them into the glass of blender and crush.
Add the water and crush again until you get a homogeneous texture. If necessary, rectify water.
Take the soup as a snack at any time of the day to purify the body and keep cravings at bay. To know more: This cold soup is quick to prepare and has great benefits for the body. Perhaps the best-known property of the apple is its intestinal regulatory action. If we eat it raw and with skin, it is useful to treat constipation, since this way we take advantage of its richness in insoluble fiber present in the skin, which stimulates the intestinal activity and helps to keep the intestinal muscles in shape. Also, green apples are one of the largest sources of flavonoids. These antioxidant compounds can stop the action of free radicals on the cells of the body. Eating raw fruits and vegetables is the healthiest option.
Nutrition:
Total Fat: 90
Carbohydrate: 11g
Fat: 3g
Protein: 4g

195.   Stuffed Zucchini

Preparation Time:15 minutes
Cooking time: 45 minutes
 Servings: 2
 Ingredients
2 small red onions - 2 small brown peppers
2 small round zucchinis
3 cloves garlic, minced
300 grams of chopped mushrooms
1 chopped carrot
2 teaspoons paprika
2 teaspoons dried marjoram
1 teaspoon dried thyme
300 grams of cooked lentils
120 ml of fried tomato
1 teaspoon sea
 Let and more to splash the vegetables Pepper
Directions:
Preheat the oven to 200 ° C.
Cut the tops of the vegetables and take out the interiors with a spoon. Chop the interiors of zucchini and onions.
Heat a pan over medium-high heat and add the inside of the onions, garlic, and a water jet (you can use oil). Once poached, add the mushrooms and fry until golden brown. Add the carrot and the inside of the zucchini. Fry until soft and the liquid have evaporated.
Add the paprika and herbs and fry a few seconds to release the aroma. Add the lentils, fried tomatoes, salt, and pepper and cook a few minutes so that the flavors are mixed.
Season the interiors of the empty vegetables and fill with the lentils. Place them on a tray and return their covers—Bake 45 to 60 minutes or until easily punctured with a knife.
Take a view from time to time and if the covers start to burn or remove or cover with silver paper.
Let cool a few minutes before serving.
Nutrition:
Total Fat: 170 Carbohydrate: 8g Fat: 12g Protein: 8g

196.   Pumpkins with Quinoa

Preparation Time: 5 minutes
Cooking time: 20 minutes
Servings: 2
Ingredients
2 medium violin pumpkins
1 cup of quinoa
1 cup cooked chickpeas
2 tbsp. of pine nuts
2 tbsp. of blueberries
Dried reds
A few sprigs of parsley
4 tbsp. extra virgin olive oil
Salt
Pepper
1 teaspoon turmeric
1 cup. fresh spinach
Directions:
Cut the pumpkins in half lengthwise and, with the help of a spoon, remove the seeds. Place them in a baking dish lined with sulfurized paper and cook in the preheated oven at 200 degrees for 1 hour. Click with a knife to check that they are well cooked, remove from the oven and let it temper.
Wash the quinoa. In a saucepan, boil plenty of saltwater and add the quinoa. Cook 20 minutes, drain, and reserve. With the assistance of a spoon, empty the pumpkins, leaving a little pulp so as not to break the peel.
Heat a pan with olive oil; add the chopped pumpkin pulp, quinoa, cooked and drained chickpeas, pine nuts, cranberries, and chopped parsley—season with Salt, Pepper, and a little turmeric. Sauté a couple of minutes and, finally, add fresh spinach. Sauté one more minute and remove from heat. Fill the pumpkins with the mixture, sprinkle with a pinch of turmeric and serve.
Nutrition:
Total Fat: 129
Carbohydrate: 23.4g
Fat: 3.3g
Protein: 4.3g

197.   Pea salad, gourmet peas, grapefruit

Preparation Time: 20 minutes
Cooking time: 10 minutes
Servings: 6
Ingredients
1 pink grapefruit
4 cups shelled peas
1 cup gourmet peas
2 fresh onions with the stem
1 tray of sprouted seeds
1 drizzles of olive oil
1 dash of apple cider vinegar
1 tbsp. old-fashioned mustard
Seeds sesame toasted
Directions:
Peel the grapefruit and collect the flesh (without the white skin), as well as the juice.
Steam peas 3-4 minutes and gourmet peas a little more.
Mix the mustard in a salad bowl with the grapefruit juice, olive oil, vinegar, salt, and Pepper. Add the chopped onions with the stem, the vegetables, and the grapefruit flesh. Mix well, sprinkle with sesame and sprinkle with sprouted seeds.
Nutrition:
Total Fat: 400
Carbohydrate: 3 g
Fat: 40g
Protein: 11g

198.   Indian pea dip

Preparation Time: 10 minutes
Servings: 4
Ingredients
1 cup frozen peas
2 tbsp. of coriander
2 tbsp. of mint
1 chopped green pepper
2 organic limes
2 tbsp. of coconut cream
Salt pepper
Directions:
Cover 200 g of frozen peas with boiling water.
In a bowl, mix 2 tsp. Coriander and 2 tsp. Minced mint, chopped green Pepper, zest of 2 organic limes, juice of 1 lime, 2 tsp. Coconut cream, salt, and Pepper.
Mash the drained peas; mix them with the rest of the ingredients.
Nutrition:
Total Fat: 93
Carbohydrate: 9 g
Fat: 5g
Protein: 4g

199.   Millet Veggie Kale Paupiettes, Apple Pear Chutney

Preparation Time: 40 minutes

Cooking time: 75 minutes

Servings: 4

Ingredients
1 large cabbage kale - 4 cups millet or quinoa - 2 onions.2 cloves of garlic
2 multicolored carrots - 1 celery stalk - 2 sprigs of parsley
1/2 teaspoon curry powder - 4 tbsp.. of olive oil
hot vegetable or poultry broth
For the chutney
2 pears - 2 apples.1 onion. - The juice of 1 orange
1 tbsp. peeled and grated ginger
3 tbsp. of apple cider vinegar
2 tbsp. soup sugar cane
Directions:
Blanch the 12 largest cabbage leaves for 10 minutes in a casserole dish of salted boiling water. Drain them; pass them under cold water, then remove the central rib if it is thick.

Rinse the millet or quinoa, and then cook it for 8 minutes in boiling salted water. Drain it. Chop the parsley. Peel and chop the onions. Peel, peel, and chop the garlic cloves. Peel the carrots and cut them into brunoised. Chop the celery. Heat the olive oil in a Dutch oven and brown the onions, garlic, carrots, celery, and curry for 15 minutes over low heat. Add salt and Pepper. Mix the quinoa or millet and the vegetables.

Preheat the oven to 180 ° / the 6. Stuff the cabbage leaves with the cereal-vegetable mixture and form small packages. Tie them. Store the paupiettes in a baking dish, drizzle with broth and cook for 20 to 30 minutes with small simmers. Lower the temperature if the lids start to color.

For the chutney, peel and seed the pears and apples. Cut them into pieces. Peel and chop the onion. Gather all the ingredients inside a saucepan and cook for about 20 minutes. Let cool.

Serve the paupiettes with a little cooking broth and the chutney aside.
Nutrition:
Total Fat: 60 Carbohydrate: 15 g Fat: 0g Protein: 4g

200.   Broad Beans, Peas, Gourmet Peas, and Mint

Preparation Time: 30 minutes
Cooking time: 30 minutes
Servings: 4
Ingredients
peas - beans - 4 cups gourmet peas
sugar
25 cl + 1/2 teaspoon (s) Coffee white balsamic vinegar
4 tbsp. pea sprouts
4 tbsp. sagebrush
1 onion withers
1 cl olive oil
1 bunch of mint 60 cl milk
Directions:
Shell the peas and beans. Bring 1.5 l of salted water to a boil in a saucepan, add the pea pods and cook for 10 minutes. Remove them with a skimmer. Add the peas to the broth, and then cook for 3 to 4 minutes. Take out the peas with a skimmer and cool them in ice water.
Mix 2/3 of the peas with 50 cl of cooking broth to obtain a soup. Reserve 1/3 of the peas and the remaining cooking broth.
Place the chopped mint in a saucepan, add the milk, and bring to the boil. Remove from the heat, let steep for 30 minutes, filter, and set aside. Dip the gourmet peas 2 to 3 minutes in a saucepan of boiling salted water, then the beans 1 to 2 minutes. Let them cool in ice water. Remove the skin from the beans.
Reduce 25 cl of balsamic vinegar until you get a syrupy juice. In the reserved cooking broth, heat the beans, the 1/3 peas, and the gourmet peas for 2 to 3 minutes.
Heat and froth the mint milk. Heat the pea soup; add a few sprouts of peas and sagebrush, season with olive oil, and the rest of the white balsamic vinegar.
In a deep plate, pour the pea soup, add the beans, gourmet peas, and drained peas. Add the chopped sweet onion, the sugar, the rest of the pea and sagebrush sprouts, the reduced vinegar, and the frothed mint milk.
Nutrition:
Total Fat: 255 Carbohydrate: 14 g Fat: 16g Protein: 10g

201.   Broccoli, Zucchini & Onions Soup: Super Healthy Recipe

Preparation Time: 15 minutes
Servings: 4
Ingredients
- 4 tbsp. broccoli
- ½ courgette
- ½ red onion
- 1 C. Tablespoon of coconut oil
- 4 cups of water
- 1 bouillon-cube with herbs

Directions:
Cut the red onion and zucchini into small pieces.
Then cut the broccoli florets.
Heat the coconut oil inside a pan and fry the red onion for about 3 minutes.
Then cook the zucchini for 5 minutes.
Add the broccoli florets, water, and bouillon cube. Simmer on low heat for 4 minutes.
Reduce everything to the blender until you get a creamy soup.
This broccoli, zucchini, and onion soup can be served immediately or reheated as you wish. Enjoy your meal!

Nutrition:
Total Fat: 115
Carbohydrate: 17 g
Fat: 0g
Protein:5g

Conclusion

In this early phase, a thinking approach is to look and feel the health effects on both your body and clothing and how your clothes match less snugly than simply concentrating on your body weight.

Feed the juices out all day long instead of getting them so close together. Take the juices at least one or two hours before and after meals, and eat no later than 7 p.m.

Although the early stage of juicing and fasting is ideal for those who might want to lose a little weight rapidly, the Sirtfood diet's overall goal is to include nutritious foods in your diet to improve your well-being and immune system. There's one more important goal, though. Although the first seven days can sound incredibly challenging, the longer-term approach will work for everybody.

You will start the fat burning while enjoying your daily favorites by concentrating on incorporating Sirtfood rich ingredients into your everyday meals. It is an eating program and will continue to provide results for a long period.

There are over 200 recipes all of which can help you along every step of your journey to reach your goal. Whether your favorite recipe is No-Bake Triple Berry Mini-Tarts, Chicken with Veggies, Buckwheat noodles with salmon and rocket, Kale & Cucumber Smoothie, Scrambled eggs, or Mozzarella Cauliflower Bars, you are sure to find a number of dishes that you love.
Whether you start out following the Sirt diet to the letter or simply experimenting and enjoying the dishes, you are sure to experience benefits and fall in love with food all over again. What are you waiting for? With just a little effort and time in the kitchen, you can get on your way to success.
The Sirt Food diet is a type of diet, it undoubtedly has significant advantages, it can make you lose weight and maintain muscle mass, but as mentioned above, it is not the only one.
The diet helps us to continue eating many foods, which in other diet forbids. However, as explained, this does not mean being able to eat without control. Indeed, we must follow an extremely strict protocol. With this, I do not want to discourage you, but only to make you realize that there are other ways,

which can lead to equally valid results. It should be stressed, however, that the Sirt Food diet is considered safe; the side effects are minimal and temporary. Clearly, like all approaches, they provide contraindications in some pathological cases.

Part of making healthy food choices time to set yourself up for success. It's always difficult to make a healthy choice when there isn't healthy food offered to you!

Keeping your kitchen stocked with healthy food is the first step to success, so it has some practical grocery store ideas that you can run in and get when you do not have any food left in your home!

Even with a hectic schedule, you can still ensure that you are eating healthy, healthy meals. By putting in a bit of Directions: you can ensure that you and your family take pleasure in healthy foods that support your lifestyle and your objectives.

With a little perseverance and Directions: it is possible to prepare and consume healthy, wholesome meals at supper time. Without taking much time from your schedule, you can repair these meals for yourself, some buddies, or for your whole household.

Printed in Great Britain
by Amazon